GESTATIONAL DIABETES - CAUSES, DIAGNOSIS AND TREATMENT

Edited by **Luis Sobrevia**

Gestational Diabetes - Causes, Diagnosis and Treatment
http://dx.doi.org/10.5772/46133
Edited by Luis Sobrevia

Contributors

Luis Sobrevia, Begum, Gregory Edward Rice, Murray Mitchell, Carlos Salomon, Keith Ashman, Sebastián Illanes, Alexander Emeakpor Omu, Elaine Christine Dantas Moisés, Fabian Pardo, Andrea Leiva, Camila Diez De Medina, Carlos Escudero

Published by InTech
Janeza Trdine 9, 51000 Rijeka, Croatia

Notice

Publishing Process Manager Ana Pantar
Technical Editor InTech DTP team
Cover InTech Design team

Additional hard copies can be obtained from orders@intechopen.com

Gestational Diabetes - Causes, Diagnosis and Treatment , Edited by Luis Sobrevia
p. cm.
ISBN 978-953-51-1077-4

For EU product safety concerns:
IN TECH d.o.o., Prolaz Marije Krucifikse Kozulić 3, 51000 Rijeka, Croatia,
info@intechopen.com or visit our website at intechopen.com.

Meet the editor

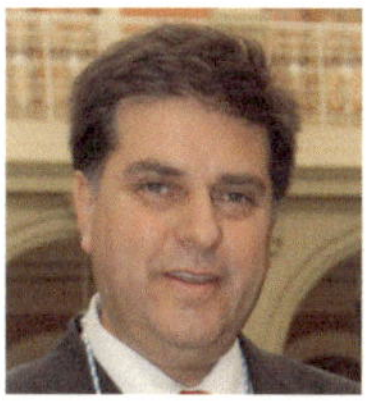

Professor Luis Sobrevia is a biologist holding MSc in Physiology from Universidad de Concepción (Chile), PhD in Biomedical Sciences from King´s College London (UK). He is Professor at the Faculty of Medicine of the Pontificia Universidad Católica de Chile and Honorary Professor at the University of Queensland Centre for Clinical Research (UQCCR), Australia. His research interest is vascular physiology focused on cellular and molecular mechanisms regulating gene expression, transcripts and protein products associated with plasma membrane transporters and receptors in micro and macrovascular endothelium of the human placenta under pathological conditions, including preeclampsia and gestational diabetes.

Contents

Preface

Gestational diabetes (GD) is a syndrome characterized by glucose intolerance with onset or first recognition during pregnancy. This definition is widely and properly used in clinical terms. Something that at present is not well defined is the potential consequence of GD in the fetal development and increased postnatal risks. The, by now, clearer concept regarding health alterations in adulthood due to an abnormal intrauterine environment is something that indeed requires considering in order to better understand the consequences of human diseases of pregnancy. GD is one of the syndromes associated with altered phenotype at birth. Certainly, a proper management of these patients must be considered in order to diminish the health risk for the mother and the fetus.

In this book the contributors have compiled several aspects that should be considered in pregnancies with GD. The book is divided into two sections: (a) GD Patient Care and Considerations, and (b) Cell and Molecular Mechanisms Behind this Syndrome. In the first section (Chapter 1), **Professor M.R. Begum** (AKM Medical College, Dhaka, Bangladesh) proposes several management recommendations for a better comprehension of the diseases in pregnancy and its consequences. In this review, it is proposed that pregnancy progresses with changes in maternal carbohydrate occur and the placental hormones act as contrainsulin factor leading to insulin resistance with a final increase in insulin secretion. When this physiological compensation is inadequate, then GD develops. Unfortunately, we do not have tools for an early diagnosis of GD, or, even more importantly, a protocol that allows prevention of GD, but as soon as this syndrome is diagnosed or recognized management is required. GD ends in a sort of associated alterations in the mother (eg., preeclampsia, type 2 diabetes mellitus (DMT2) and others) and the fetus (eg., congenital anomaly, macrosomia and others). Thus, management of this syndrome aims mainly at maintaining euglycemia, preventing obstetrical complications and reaching optimal timing and appropriate mode of delivery. This chapter presents discussion which addresses suggestions for the management of patients including counselling, the role of nutrition and/or insulin therapy, or pharmacological treatment including oral antiadiabetic agents such as glybenclamide and metformin. In Chapter 2, **Professor E.C. Dantas Moisés** (University of São Paulo, Brazil) proposes a multidisciplinary care of pregnant women with the diagnosis of GD. Complementing the previous chapter, this chapter includes non-pharmacological strategies to improve maternal and perinatal outcomes. Several aspects are touched in this concept, including nutrition. The chapter highlights the need for healthy eating habits according to the nutritional needs, physical activity as a strategy for prevention, and professional support from psychologists, nurses, social workers, and multidisciplinary groups. It is proposed that prenatal care of women is certainly required and that it is essential to provide information about the pathophysiology and prognosis of diabetes mellitus, either pregestational or gestational at this stage. Indeed, the United Nations (UN) Secretary General of World Health Organization (WHO) organized a special session of the UN General Assembly (2011) to address the control and prevention of non-communicable chronic diseases, presently the main cause of death and loss of health, which highlighted the importance of the health status of future mothers (i.e., pre-pregnancy) and its consequences on the health of fetus and the newborn. There is certainly a need for this and more research centres formed by multi and interdisciplinary groups should consider this concept.

In the second section of this book, five different contributions are presented referring to cell and molecular mechanisms behind the genesis or consequences of GD. The contribution by **Dr C. Salomon** (University of Queensland, Australia) **and colleagues** (Chapter 3) explores the importance of new mechanisms of communication between the trophoblasts and other cell types in the placenta in GD. One of the mechanisms discussed in this chapter is the capacity of the trophoblasts to release nanovesicles including exosomes, and its potential putative utility in the diagnosis of disease onset and treatment monitoring, including GD. The authors discuss the biogenesis and role of placental exosomes as a mechanism to engage in local cell-to-cell communication and/or distal interactions as release of placental exosomes into biological fluids and their transport to a remote site of action. The central idea behind this proposal is that placental-derived exosomes may be of utility as diagnostic markers of GD in asymptomatic pregnant women. A conclusion of this review leads us to ask whether nanovesicles released from the trophoblasts will modulate the function of endothelial cells of the human placenta, especially in GD. In the section reviewed by **Dr E. Guzmán-Gutiérrez and colleagues** (Pontificia Universidad Católica de Chile) (Chapter 4) a link between the biological effects of insulin in the placenta vasculature and the endogenous nucleoside adenosine is proposed. GD is also a syndrome that occurs with maternal and fetal insulin resistance and adenosine modulates the biological action of insulin on L-arginine/nitric oxide (NO) signalling pathway (the L-arginine/NO signalling pathway) in human umbilical vein endothelial cells (HUVECs) from normal pregnancies. Thus, the authors propose that GD associates with endothelial dysfunction in the fetoplacental macro and microcirculation and further suggest the involvement of A2A adenosine receptors and insulin receptors as a mechanism explaining the increase of NO synthesis (i.e., potential modulation of the reported ALANO pathway (Adenosine/L-Arginine/Nitric Oxide) (San Martín & Sobrevia, *Placenta,* 2006). It is also discussed that insulin has a dual effect regarding modulation of L-arginine transport and NO synthesis in HUVECs. This is explained by a potential differential expression of insulin receptor isoforms A (IR-A) and IR-B in normal and GD pregnancies, as confirmed in recent studies in HUVECs (Westermeier et al, *Diabetes,* 2011) and human placental microvascular endothelial cells (Salomon et al, *PLoS ONE,* 2012). In fact, since insulin effects are dependent on activation of adenosine receptors in several cell types, including HUVECs (Guzmán-Gutiérrez et al, *PLoS ONE,* 2012), it is suggested that a differential regulation of expression and/or activity of insulin receptor isoforms by activation of adenosine receptors could be used as a strategy to improve GD deleterious effects in the mother and the fetus. In these terms, **Professor A. Omu** (Kuwait University, Kuwait) (Chapter 5) proposes that a complementary action is required, including mechanisms and consequences of alterations in lipid metabolism during pregnancy, which associates diabetes in pregnancy with obese patients. Furthermore, inflammation-induced insulin resistance is also reviewed in this chapter and a potential correlation with the epidemic of obesity is proposed (Pardo et al, *J Diab Metab,* 2012). Professor Omu also highlights the need for genetic studies to identify subjects with candidate genes for diabetes and epigenetic factors that may affect gene expression and predisposition to inflammation. Early recognition and management of women predisposed to develop diabetes is crucial for prevention or delaying insulin resistance and development of glucose intolerance. The epidemiology, genetics and immunological basis of GD, the role of lipid metabolism and lipid peroxidation, oxidative stress on antioxidant gene expression and other inflammatory cytokines, as well as the role of risk factors such as obesity and adipokynes, proinflammatory cytokines, and the role of intervention strategies in the prevention of progression of GD to DMT2 and maternal effects of GD is extensively reviewed and proposed in this review. In the chapter by **Dr A. Leiva and colleagues** (Pontificia Universidad Católica de Chile) (Chapter 6) the role of maternal plasma cholesterol levels in pregnancy is analysed. Maternal supraphysiological hypercholesterolemia (MSPH) occurs with pathologies including GD. Since GD is also associated with endothelial dysfunction of the placenta mainly triggered by dyslipidemia, it is proposed that MSPH could play a role in this phenomenon since dyslipidemia is a risk factor in developing endothelial dysfunction and atherosclerosis. The main topic of this review highlights the fact that atherogenesis, a clinical complication commonly appearing in adults, might begin in fetal life with similar factors altered at the mother, the fetus and the placenta. Another proposal is the fact that umbilical veins could potentially be altered by MSPH. This is rather new in the literature and the mechanisms are unknown; however, umbilical vein as a model of fetal arteries (i.e., carrying fetal blood rich in oxygen) could represent a biological substrate for studying the mechanisms associated with fetal atherosclerosis biogenesis. The authors describe alterations in the L-arginine/NO pathway and the role of arginases in this phenomenon. These mechanisms have not been evaluated in GD occuring with hypercholesterolemia (Leiva et al, *Exp Diab Res,* 2011). Finally, the review by **Dr C. Escudero** (Universidad del Bío-Bío, Chile) **and colleagues** (Chapter 7) supports several aspects of the information described in previous chapters and includes general and specific ideas regarding dysfunction of the endothelial cells from the microvasculature of the human placenta in GD. This review summarizes the available literature focused on the role of feto-placental endothelial dysfunction as the possible main factor in the generation of short-term complication during GD and certainly speculates how it may program the response of the fetus to a 'GD environment'. Several aspects are put in a well coordinated description of mechanisms, anatomy and histology of the placenta, changes in blood flow, the role of oxidative stress, with a description of placental angiogenesis involving adenosine (Escudero et al, *Biofactors,* 2012).

A final general remark of chapters in this book is, in fact, that GD is a syndrome caused by a not well-understood multifactor mechanism. However, common strategies seem to be key in the understanding of the syndrome, i.e., endothelial dysfunction and the role of other placenta cells such as trophoblasts. A proper and knowledge-based management of the syndrome for the well being of the mother and the fetus is fully needed. In addition, pre-pregnancy and antenatal screening of women is required. This is not only to improve the management and outcome of the pregnancy but also to optimize life-long health and well being, considering the inter-generational consequences. Thus, pre-pregnancy health and nutrition are key conditioning factors for fetal development and the health of the newborn, which are, in turn, major determinants of adult chronic diseases.

Professor Luis Sobrevia
Cellular and Molecular Physiology Laboratory (CMPL)
Division of Obstetrics and Gynaecology
School of Medicine, Faculty of Medicine
Pontificia Universidad Católica de Chile
Santiago, Chile.
Honorary Professor
The University of Queensland Centre for Clinical Research
Herston, QLD, Australia.

Acknowledgments
The contents of this book have been made possible thanks to the generous contributions of all authors, who have made a dedicated effort to compile information focused on the central topic of the book. Special thanks are given to the Division of Obstetrics and Gynecology of the School of Medicine of the Faculty of Medicine, Pontificia Universidad Católica de Chile for the support to proceed with this project. Secretarial assistance (Mrs Ninoska Muñoz) in the editorial process of these reviews was partially provided from Fondo Nacional de Desarrollo Científico y Tecnológico (FONDECYT 1110977) and Programa de Investigación Interdisciplinario (PIA) from Comisión Nacional de Investigación en Ciencia y Tecnología (CONICYT, Anillos ACT-73) (Chile).

Section 1

GD Patient Care and Considerations

Chapter 1

GDM: Management Recommendations During Pregnancy

Mosammat Rashida Begum

Additional information is available at the end of the chapter

http://dx.doi.org/10.5772/55467

1. Introduction

Gestational diabetes mellitus (GDM) is currently defined as any degree of glucose intolerance with onset or first recognition during current pregnancy [1-4]. Pregnancy induces progressive changes in maternal carbohydrate metabolic process. As pregnancy advances insulin resistance and diabetogenic stress due to placental contra-insulin hormones necessitate compensatory increase in insulin secretion. When this compensatory mechanism fails due to pancreatic β cells inadequacy gestational diabetes develops. GDM affects 1-2% of all pregnancies. In majority of patients it is mild and can be adequately controlled with diet alone but a minority will require antidiabetogenic agents like glyburide or insulin.

Abnormalities of carbohydrate metabolism occur during pregnancy lead to glucose intolerance. Due to diabetogenic effect of pregnancy about 3-5% of all pregnant women show glucose intolerance and approximately 90% of these women have GDM. Majority of these women will have normal carbohydrate tolerance after delivery. However, 50% of women with GDM will develop type 2 DM later in their life. Asian women are ethnically more prone to develop glucose intolerance compared to other ethnic groups. Due to many adverse effects of GDM on mother and foetus early diagnosis and appropriate management is essential for improved outcome of pregnancy.

2. How does pregnancy cause carbohydrate intolerance?

As pregnancy advances it causes

a. Increased insulin resistance due to

1. Antagonistic effect of increased production of human placental lactogen
2. Anti-insulin effect of increased production of placental cortisol, oestriol and progesterone.
3. Increased insulin catabolism by placental and renal insulinase [5]

b. Increased blood glucose level because

1. Mother utilized fat for her caloric requirements and saves glucose for her foetus.

As a result of these physiological changes the normal blood sugar pattern in pregnant woman is Fasting - 65 ± 9mg/dl, non fasting - 80 ± 10 mg/dl, postprandial - 140 ± 10 mg/dl [6].

3. Adverse effects of GDM

Carbohydrate intolerance during pregnancy or GDM causes significant increases in foetal and maternal morbidity. The maternal consequences are

- Preeclampsia: 10-25% of all pregnant diabetes.
- Infection: High incidence of chorioamnionitis and postnatal endometritis.
- Polyhydramnios
- Postpartum bleeding- High incidence due to exaggerated uterine distension.
- Caeserean section: High incidence due to fetal cause.
- Delayed wound healing or wound dehiscence if GDM is not controlled
- Long term effect is type 2 DM.

Fetuses are much more affected than mothers. The fetal consequences are

- Congenital anomaly: It is associated with poor glycemic control and end organ damage.
- Macrosomia: It is defined as a birth weight greater than or equal to 4000 g. Incidence is 17-29% of pregnancies with GDM as compared with 10% in the nondiabetic population [7].
- Hypoglycemia The incidence of neonatal hypoglycemia is greater in GDM than normal pregnancies [8].
- Hypocalcaemia
- Hyaline membrane disease
- Apnea and bradycardia
- Traumatic delivery: The incidence of shoulder dystocia with brachial plexus damage and clavicular fractures are increased in neonates of women with GDM [9]
- Stillbirth

The neonatal morbidity is assessed by a composite outcome that includes stillbirth, neonatal macrosomia or LGA, neonatal hypoglycemia, erythrocytosis and hyperbilirubenemia. Langer et al found composite morbidity in 59% of untreated GDM, 18% of treated GDM and in 11% of non-diabetic subjects [9]. The most common complication was macrosomia which affected 46% and 19% of the newborns from untreated and treated mothers with GDM respectively.

4. How to diagnose GDM?

To diagnose GDM first of all screening is done to detect the potential cases for GDM. A number of screening procedures and diagnostic criteria are followed in different countries like American Diabetes Association (ADA), World Health Organization (WHO), Canadian Diabetes Association (CDA), National Diabetes Data Group (NDDG) and Australian criteria. Two types of screening methods are adopted by different populations. In selective screening, only high risk populations are screened and in universal screening, all pregnant women are included. American Diabetes Association (ADA) recommends screening of selective (High risk) population. But compared to selective screening, universal screening for GDM detects more cases and improves maternal and neonatal prognosis [10]. So universal screening appears to be the most reliable and desired method for detection of GDM [11].

ADA screening: ADA recommends two step screening.

Step1:- A 50 gm glucose challenge test (GCT) is used for screening without regard to the time of last meal or time of the day [12)

Step 2:-If 1hour GCT value is more than 140 mg/dl, 100 g oral glucose tolerance test (OGTT) is recommended and plasma glucose is estimated at 0,1,2 and 3 hours. GDM is diagnosed if any 2 values meet or exceed fasting plasma glucose (FPG) >95 mg/dl, 1 hour postparandial glucose (PG)> 180 mg/dl, 2 hour PG> 155 mg/dl and 3 hour PG >140 mg/dl. But drawback of this method is that, the glycaemic control cut-off was originally validated against the future risk of mother only and on the foetal outcome [13]. Other problems are the number of blood samples requirement is more, 1 for screening and 4 for 3 hour OGTT to confirm the diagnosis. Moreover, patients have to visit the antenatal clinic at least on two occasions for diagnosis leading to their inconvenience.

WHO procedure: To standardize the diagnosis of GDM the World Health Organization (WHO) recommends using a 2 hour OGTT with a threshold plasma glucose concentration of greater than 140 mg/dl at 2 hours, similar to that of impaired glucose tolerance (IGT) in non pregnant state [14]. WHO procedure also was not based on maternal and foetal outcome but probably the criteria was recommended for its easy adaptability in clinical practice. WHO criteria of 2 hour plasma glucose ≥140 mg/dl identifying a large number of cases may have greater potential for prevention of GDM [15].

A single test procedure for diagnosis of GDM: All the diagnostic criteria require the women to be fasting. For successful implementation of universal screening the procedure should not impose any restriction. So a single test 2-hours after 75 g glucose in a non-fasting state irrespective of last meal can make the diagnostic procedure simple, feasible and economical. It serves as both screening and diagnostic procedure, causes least disturbance to a pregnant woman's routine activities and avoids the inconvenience of fasting in a pregnant woman. It was found that there was no significant difference in PG level between 75g glucose testing in fasting and non-fasting state, irrespective of last meal timing [16]. Performing this test procedure in the non-fasting state is rational, as glucose concentration are affected little by the time since last meal in a normal glucose tolerant woman, whereas meal timing affects in a woman with GDM [17] The non-fasting 2-h post 75 g glucose correctly identified subjects with GDM [18] and strongly predict adverse outcome for the mother and her offspring [19]. Thus, the single test procedure performed irrespective of the last meal timing is seems to be a more rational and patient friendly approach.

Diagnosis	**Fasting plasma glucose (FPG) (Mg/dl)**	**2-hour plasma glucose (PG) (Mg/dl)**
Normal glucose tolerance (NGT)	<100	<140
Impaired fasting glucose (IFG)	100-125	
Impaired glucose tolerance (IGT)		140-199
Diabetes mellitus (DM)	≥126	≥200

Table 1. Classification of glucose intolerance by 75gm 2 hour oral glucose tolerance test(OGTT)

5. When to screen in pregnancy?

Increasing maternal carbohydrate intolerance in pregnant woman without GDM is associated with adverse maternal and foetal outcome [20]. By following the usual recommendation for screening between 24-28 weeks of gestation many early onset of GDM and pre pregnant unidentified diabetes mellitus (DM) can be missed, which may adversely affect foetal outcome. Seshiah et al detected 16.3% glucose intolerance within 16 weeks of pregnancy [21]. Other two studies reported about 40% to 66% of women with GDM can be detected early during pregnancy [22,23]. Nahum et al suggested that the ideal period to screen for GDM is around 16 weeks of gestation and even earlier in high-risk groups with a history of foetal wastage [23]. GDM diagnosis may not be missed by screening around 24-28 weeks of gestation but a substantial number of pregnant women who develop GDM in the earlier weeks of gestation are likely to have delayed diagnosis and may not receive appropriate medical care. So it is safe to screen for GDM during early weeks of pregnancy as by early detection of glucose intolerance during pregnancy and adequate care to the antenatal women a good foetal outcome can be achieved similar to that of normal glucose tolerance (NGT) pregnant women [24, 25]. If a woman is found to have normal glucose tolerance test in the first trimester, she should be tested for GDM around 24th -28th weeks and around 32nd-34th weeks and also in later weeks if necessary, particularly when rapid weight gain occurs or foetal macrosomia is suspected [26].

It has been suggested that women at high risk should be screened as soon as pregnancy is confirmed [27].

6. High risk GDM

Gestational diabetes is a complication during pregnancy which affects both mother and foetus. From foetal point of view adverse affects are sometimes severe and fatal. Some GDM patients are at higher risk for complications than others. High risk GDM patients are those who have the

- History of stillbirth, neonatal death and foetal macrosomia in previous pregnany
- Maternal obesity and hypertension
- Development of oligohydramnios, polyhydramnios, preeclampsia
- Inadequate metabolic control by diet alone.

Women at high risk should be identified soon after the diagnosis is made, because they need meticulous management to prevent such complications, need antepartum foetal surveillance testing and may require delivery before their expected date of delivery.

7. Management strategies

To prevent maternal and fetal complications treatment at appropriate time is necessary. Early detection of glucose intolerance during pregnancy and instillation of treatment at earliest state can prevent the complications and a good fetal outcome can be achieved.

So, aim of management is to

- Maintain euglycemia
- Prevent obstetrical complications
- Fix optimal time and appropriate mode of delivery

Management includes

1. Counseling of the patient

It is important to counsel the patient with GDM about the condition and its management, so that they can acquire a clear understanding of the characteristics and demands be emphasized on

1. the importance of exercise and diet control

2. importance of blood glucose control

3. self monitoring of blood glucose

4. identification and treatment of hypoglycemia.

2. Treatment of blood glucose control

The fundamental objective of the care of every insulin dependent pregnant diabetic is control of blood glucose to a desirable level for good fetal outcome. The aim is to maintain the fasting glucose level between 80-90mg/dl and 2 hours postprandial glucose level between 110-129mg/dl.

7.1. Medical Nutrition Therapy (MNT)

Dieting is an important step for blood glucose control. But pregnancy needs extra calories for growth and development of fetus. So GDM patients need strict maintenance of diet to maintain adequate calories without affecting blood glucose level to have a healthy baby. The concept of dietary management of the GDM or any other diabetic pregnant woman is that a healthy diet for them is not different from a healthy diet for any other non-diabetic pregnant woman. Patients should know that carbohydrate containing food increase blood glucose levels above normal limits and that persistently abnormal elevation of the blood glucose levels are harmful both for mother and foetus. So to prevent abnormal glucose levels a food plan should be made to maintain adequate calories without affecting blood glucose levels. Patient needs to understand the quantity or servings of carbohydrate present in her meals and snacks and the effect of different types of carbohydrate on her blood glucose levels.

The meal pattern should provide adequate calories and nutrients to meet the needs of pregnancy. The expected weight gain during pregnancy is 300-400g/week and total weight gain is 10-12 kg by term. So the meal plan aims to provide sufficient calories to sustain adequate nutrition for the mother and foetus and to avoid excess weight gain and postprandial hyperglycemia. Calculation of daily caloric intake is based on body weight, age, physical activities and gestational age. Approximately 30-40 kcal/kg and an increment of 300 kcal/day above the basal requirement are needed in 2nd and 3rd trimester. For majority of women with GDM the optional total daily caloric intake will be between 2000 and 2500 cal/day. The total caloric intake is split into three meals and one to three snacks depending on the patient's habit. In a non-diabetic woman the peaking of the plasma glucose is high after breakfast due to "Dawn phenomenon"and the insulin secretion also matches the glycemic excursion that occurs with the meal [28]. But GDM mothers have deficiency in first phase insulin secretion leads to increased postprandial glucose level after heavy breakfast. To avoid the postprandial plasma glucose peaking with breakfast, it can be split into two halves and consuming these portions with a two-hour gap. By this, the undue peak in plasma glucose levels after ingestion of the total quantity of breakfast at one time is avoided.

The total daily caloric allowance should be distributed among the different foods groups in such a way that approximately 40-50% of the calories come from complex carbohydrate. The carbohydrate component of the diet should be distributed as 10-15% at breakfast, 20-30% at lunch and 30-40% at dinner. Approximately 30-40% from fat and the rest from protein. Postprandial elevations of blood sugar are due almost exclusively to the carbohydrate content of the diet. So carbohydrate should be taken as small frequent meal. Growthwer et al showed the benefit of MNT is series of 1000 pregnant women in comparison to routine care. Serious complications were 1% in MNT and 4% in routine care. Macrosomia rate was 10% in MNT and 21% in routine care. There was no perinatal death in MNT group whereas 5 perinatal deaths were in routine care [29]. Benefits of MNT are

- Decreases hospital admission.
- Decrease in insulin use.
- Improved likelihood of normal foetal and placental growth.
- Reduced risk of perinatal complications specially when diagnosed and treated early

7.2. Oral antidiabetic agents

Oral hypoglycemic agents can be used to control blood glucose where nutritional therapy is failed. Two important agents are used.

Glibenclamide: Glibenclamide (Glyburide) is safe therapy for many GDM women. This drug decreases the insulin resistance and improves insulin secretion. Placental transfer of glybenclamide is negligible. Langer et al concluded that glyburide is as effective as insulin in maintaining the desired glycemic levels and resulted in a comparable outcome [30]. Only 4% of women in the glyburide group were not adequately controlled and required insulin. The usual starting dose of glyburide is 2.5 mg once or twice daily. A randomized clinical trial comparing the effect of insulin and glyburide showed equally good glycemic control and similar perinatal outcome [31]. The total daily dose may be increased up-to 20 mg if necessary. The peak plasma level occurs 2-4 hours after administration and duration of action is 10-12 hours. Women with fasting hyperglycemia but normal postprandial blood glucose may do well with a single dose of glyburide at bed time. Glyburide is a sulfonylurea and its primary mechanism of action is stimulation of the release of insulin from the storage granules of pancreatic beta cells. Secondarily it decreases insulin resistance. It is nonteratogenic and is classified as a category B drug. The main side effect of glyburide is hypoglycemia.

Metformin: Though use of metformin in pregnancy is controversial, studies shows that it can prevent the development of GDM in high risk for developing that. There were no adverse effects to fetus and mother [32, 33]. Metformin trial in gestational diabetes found that in women with GDM, metformin was not associated with increased peinatal complications as compared with insulin [34]. Usual dose is 500 mg to 1500 mg daily in divided doses. Metformin appears to suppress hepatic glucose uptake and decreases intestinal absorption of glucose. It is also a category B drug and it does not cause hypoglycemia. More studies needed before recommendation for routine use in pregnancy.

7.3. Insulin therapy

Once diagnosis is made, nutrition therapy is advised. If it fails oral antidiabetic agents can be tried. If oral agents failed to acheive FPG of ≤ 5.0 mmol/L and 2-h postprandial glucose level of ≤ 6.7 mmol/L insulin is to be started. The aim is to maintain the postprandial peak plasma glucose level of ≤ 6.7 mmol/L. Human insulin is the insulin of choice for the first time. Most patients require a mixture of intermediate (NPH) and regular (short acting) insulin twice daily. It is preferable to start with premix insulin (mixture of NPH and regular insulin) of any brand. Usually women with GDM do not require >20 unit insulin per day for glycemic control [35]. Recommended dosing schedule is two thirds of the total insulin dose is to be given in the morning and remainder before dinner. The morning dose should be two thirds NPH and one third short acting insulin and the pre-dinner dose should be equal parts NPH and short acting insulin. However, dose schedule requires modification according to patent's BMI, glucose level and life style.

Insulin analogue: If postprandial glucose is still not under control, rapid acting insulin analogue is to be considered. Rapid acting insulin analogues (Aspart-Novorapid, Lispro-Humalog) have been found to be safe and effective during pregnancy. Pregestational diabetic women during pregnancy may require high dose of insulin. A few may require multiple-daily injections usually given as short acting insulin before breakfast and lunch and intermediate acting insulin or premix before dinner. Insulin dose is always individualized and has to be adjusted according to need of the patient.

8. Monitoring of glycemic control:

8.1. Measuring blood glucose level

Meticulous monitoring is essential to achieve desired level of plasma glucose and to prevent post-insulin hypoglycemia. The success of treatment for a woman of GDM depends on glycemic control. Two hours postprandial blood glucose monitoring is preferable as the diagnosis of GDM is also based on two hour plasma glucose. GDM women have high post-breakfast plasma glucose level compared to post lunch and post dinner. So increased morning dose of short acting insulin is needed together with careful adjustment of meal timing and snacks to avoid hypoglycemia.

Once targeted blood glucose level is achieved woman with GDM require monitoring of both fasting and 2-h post breakfast glucose once in a month till 28th weeks of gestation. After 28th weeks blood glucose monitoring should be done fortnightly or more frequently if needed. After 32 weeks blood glucose monitoring should be done once a week till delivery. In high risk pregnancies continuous glucose monitoring may be needed to know the glycemic fluctuations and to plan proper insulin dosage.

8.2. Measuring HbA1c

A1c level is useful in monitoring the glucose control during pregnancy, but not for the day to day management. It serves as a prognostic value. In euglycemic state A1c value should be ≤6%. In early weeks of pregnancy A1c level is helpful to differentiate GDM from pre-pregnant diabetes. If A1c level is more than 6% it indicates that woman is pre GDM [36]. Though treatment approach is not changed based on A1c level.

8.3. Foetal surveillance

The management of GDM, based on the foetal growth and developmental defect if there is any. USG is the key diagnostic tool to detect developmental defect as well as to monitor the foetal growth. Low risk GDM patients who have glycemic control with diet alone and who do not develop any complications like polyhydaramnios, pre-eclampsia or macrosomia need ultrasonogram around 24 weeks of gestation and thereafter as needed. High risk GDM patients who are on insulin or oral antidiabetic agent should have antepartum foetal surveillance by ultrasonogram in every trimester. A foetal echo is a must at 24 weeks to rule out congenital defect. In last trimester biophysical profile is recommended twice in a week or weekly if foetus is at risk.

8.4. Timing of delivery

Low risk or uncomplicated GDM patients may be allowed to develop spontaneous labour and to deliver at term. There is no need to deliver before term unless there is evidence of macrosomia, polyhydarmnios, poor glycemic control or other obstetric complications like, pre-eclampsia or intrauterine growth retardation. Once the uncomplicated GDM patient reaches 40 weeks labour should be induced if cervix is ripe. If cervix is not ripe and estimated foetal weight (EFW) is >4000 gm elective caesarean section is to be done. High risk GDM patients should have their labour induced when they reach 38 weeks. Again C/S is to be done if EFW is >4000 gm. Preterm pregnancy termination may be needed in GDM with complications like pre-eclampsia, polyhydramnios, foetal compromise (less foetal movement) and uncontrolled diabetes. Glucocorticoid for 48 hours should be administered to accelerate lung maturity in preterm termination. Insulin requirement may be increased due to hyperglycemin effect of glucocorticoids. Spontaneous preterm labour is common in patient with GDM. Tocolysis in the form of magnesium sulphate or nifedipine can be used in preterm labour to delay delivery so that glucocorticoid therapy to accelerate lung maturity can be administered over 48 hours.

8.5. Management during labour

Most insulin treated GDM do not need insulin during labour and after delivery. During labour it is essential to monitor blood glucose every 2-4 hours. Upward deviations from normal are corrected with small doses of regular insulin or low dose IV insulin to maintain blood glucose between 100 and 120 mg/dl. If blood glucose is >120-140mg/dl, 4 unit insulin, if >140-180mg/dl 6 unit insulin and if >180 mg/dl 8 unit insulin is to be given in a drip of normal saline at a rate of 16-20 drops/m. Maternal capillary blood glucose is to be checked by glucometer every 1 hour and drip rate is to be adjusted. Dextrose infusion should be avoided. If it is given neutralizing dose of insulin is to be given. 1 unit insulin is needed to neutralize 2.5g glucose. So to neutralize the glucose of 1000 ml 5% dextrose saline 20 unit insulin is to be added with the drip. Drip rate is to be judged according to patient's requirement. Oral feeding is to be started as early as possible to avoid infusion of fluid. Monitoring should be done after delivery and 24 hours postpartum. Usually blood glucose level falls to baseline after delivery.

8.6. Neonatal management

A neonatologist should be present during delivery as GDM is a high risk pregnancy and there is chance of neonatal morbidity. Neonates are at risk of all complications similar to the infants born to mothers with overt diabetes [37]. Neonates should be monitored closely after delivery for respiratory distress. Capillary blood glucose should be monitored at 1, 2 and 4 hours after birth and before starting of feeding. Cut-0ff value is 2.6 mmol. Early breast feeding is strongly encouraged. If mother's blood glucose is not normalized insulin is advisable in lactating woman for good glycemic control.

9. Prevention of type 2 Diabetes Mellitus (DM)

There is increased risk of development of type 2 DM in patients of GDM [38] and incidence of type 2 DM is about 44% in patients who required insulin or OHA or onset of GDM before 24 weeks [39]. GDM may also recur in a future pregnancy and approximately 55% of patients who were obese or with macrosomic infants will have GDM in subsequent pregnancy [40]. So it is important to perform a 75 g GTT at 6-8 weeks postpartum. If found normal, GTT is repeated after 6 months and every year to assess glucose tolerance. Patients should be informed that about 40-60% of them will have overt diabetics when they are in their 5th decades. Weight loss, dietary control and exercise will obviously help to prevent overt diabetes later in life [41]. GDM has a far reaching consequence in predisposing their offsprings to glucose intolerance. Debelea et al found that more than 50% children who were born to women with GDM developed type 2 DM by the age 35 [42]. The important aspect of GDM is that the intrauterine milieu whether one of nutritional deprivation or nutritional plenty, results in foetal pancreatic development and peripheral response to insulin that may lead to adult onset GDM and type 2 DM[43]. So the timely action in all pregnant women with glucose intolerance to achieve euglycemia may prevent transmitting glucose intolerance from one generation to another [44].

GDM women are at increased risk of future type 2 diabetes mellitus and their children are also at risk of developing type 2 DM later in their life. Universal screening for GDM at early weeks of gestation can detect more cases at an early stage leading to early interventions and hence improves maternal and foetal outcome as early detection leads to early treatment and prevent complications and adverse effect to mother and foetus. A 2-hour 75g post glucose ≥7.8mml/L serves both as screening and diagnostic criteria which is a simple and economical one step procedure. Early detection and treatment of GDM can only prevent the all probable complications and the vicious cycle of transmitting glucose intolerance from generation to generation.

Author details

Mosammat Rashida Begum*

Address all correspondence to: rashida_icrc@yahoo.com

AKM Medical College, Dhaka, Bangladesh

References

[1] American Diabetes AssociationDiagnosis and classification of diabetes mellitus. Diabetes Care. (2006). Suppl 1:S, 43-8.

[2] American College of Obstetricians and Gynecologists Committee on Practice Bulletins-ObstetricsACOG Practice Bulletin. Clinical management guidelines for obstetrician-gynecologists. September (2001). replaces Technical Bulletin Number 200, December 1994). Gestational diabetes. Obstet Gynecol. 2001;, 98(30), 525-38.

[3] Metzger, B. E, & Coustan, D. R. Summary and recommendations of the Fourth International Workshop-Conference on Gestational Diabetes Mellitus. The Organizing Committee. Diabetes Care. (1998). Suppl 2:B, 161-7.

[4] Metzger, B. E, Buchanan, T. A, Coustan, D. R, De Leiva, A, Dunger, D. B, Hadden, D. R, et al. Summary and recommendations of the Fifth International Workshop-Conference on Gestational Diabetes Mellitus. Diabetes Care. (2007). Suppl 2:S, 251-60.

[5] Arias, F, Daftary, S. N, & Bhide, A. G. Practical guide to high risk pregnancy and delivery- A South Asian perspective. Elsevier, (2008). Diabetes and pregnancy, , 440-464.

[6] Cousins, L, Rigg, L, Hollingsworth, D, et al. The 24 hour excursion and diurnal rhythm of glucose, insulin and C-peptide in normal pregnancy. Am j Obstet gynecol (1980).

[7] Adams, K. L, Hongshe, L, Nelson, R. L, et al. Sequelae of unrecognized gestational diabetes. AM J Obstet Gynecol (1998). , 178, 1321-32.

[8] Garner, P, Okun, N, Keely, E, et al. A randomized controlled trial of strit glycemic control and tertiary level obstetric care versus routine obstetric care in the management of gestational diabetes: a pilot study. AM J Obstet Gynecol (1997). , 177, 190-95.

[9] Langer, O, & Yogev, . . Gestational diabetes: the consequences of not treating. AM J Obstet Gynecol 2005;192:989-97.

[10] Dorendra Singh IBidhumukhi Devi Th, Ibeyaima Devi Kh, Premchand Singh Th. Scientific Presentation Volume of the First National Conference of the DIPSI, February (2006). Chennai. 68.

[11] Shamsuddin, K, & Mahdy, Z. A. Siti Rafiaah, I.; et al. Risk factor screening for abnormal glucose tolerance in pregnancy. Int J Gynecol Obstet. (2001). , 75, 27-32.

[12] Swami, S. R, Mehetre, R, Shivane, V, Bandgar, T. R, Menon, P. S, & Shah, N. S. Prevalence of Carbohydrate Intolerance of Varying Degrees in Pregnant Females in Western India (Maharashtra)- A Hospital-based Study. J Indian Med Assoc (2008). , 106, 712-4.

[13] Divakar, H, Tyagi, S, Hosmani, P, & Manyonda, I. T. Diagnostic criteria influence prevalence rates for gestational diabetes: implications for interventions in an Indian pregnant population. Perinatology (2008). , 155-61.

[14] Beischer, N. A, Oats, J. N, Henry, O. A, Sheedy, M. T, & Walstab, J. E. Incidence and severity of gestational diabetes mellitus according to country of birth in women living in Australia. Diabetes (1991). Dec; 40 Suppl , 2, 35-8.

[15] Metzger, B. E, & Coustan, D. R. Summary and Recommendations of the Fourth International workshop-Conference on Gestational Diabetes Mellitus. Diabetes Care (1998). B, 161-167.

[16] Anjalakshi, C, Balaji, V, Balaji, M. S, et al. A single test procedure to diagnose gestational diabetes mellitus. Acta Diabetol. (2009). , 46(1), 51-4.

[17] Seshiah, V, & Balaji, V. Madhuri S Balaji, Sanjeevi CB, Green A. Gestational Diabetes Mellitus in India. JAPI (2004). , 52, 707-11.

[18] Pettitt, D. J, Bennett, P. H, Hanson, R. L, et al. Comparison of World Health Organization and National Diabetes Data Group procedures to detect abnormalities of glucose tolerance during pregnancy. Diabetes Care.(1994). , 17(11), 1264-68.

[19] Pettitt, D. J, Bennett, P. H, Saad, M. F, et al. Abnormal glucose tolerance during pregnancy in Pima Indian women: Long term effects on the offspring. Diabetes.(1991). , 40(2), 126-130.

[20] Gestational Diabetes Mellitus: American Diabetes Association- Clinical Practice Recommendations 2002; Diabetes Care 25 (1): S94-96.

[21] Seshiah, V, Balaji, V, Balaji, M. S, et al. (2007). Gestational Diabetes Mellitus manifests in all trimesters of pregnancy. Dia Res Clin Pract.2007;, 77(3), 482-4.

[22] Super, D. M, Edelberg, S. C, Philipson, E. H, et al. Diagnosis of gestational diabetes in early pregnancy. Diabetes Care.(1991). , 14(4), 288-94.

[23] Nahum, G. G, Wilson, S. B, & Stanislaw, H. Early pregnancy glucose screening for gestational diabetes mellitus. J Reprod Med.(2002). , 47(8), 656-62.

[24] Seshiah, V, Alexander, C, Balaji, V, et al. Glycemic control from early weeks of gestation and pregnancy outcome. Diabetes.(2006). Supp1):604

[25] Seshiah, V, Cynthia, A, Balaji, V, et al. Detection and care of women with gestational diabetes mellitus from early weeks of pregnancy results in birth weight of newborn babies appropriate for gestational age. Dia Res Clin Pract. (2008). , 80(2), 199-202.

[26] Franks, P. W, Looker, H. C, Kobes, S, Touger, L, Tataranni, P. A, Hanson, R. L, et al. Gestational Glucose tolerance and risk of type 2 diabetes in Young Pima Indian Offspring. Diabetes. (2006). Feb; , 55(2), 460-65.

[27] Gestational diabetes mellitusAmerican Diabetes Association. Diabetes Care (2003). suppl 1) 5103-5105.

[28] Polonsky, K. S, Given, B. D, & Van Cauter, E. Twenty four hour profiles and pulsatile patterns of insulin secretion in normal and obese subjects. J Clin Invest.(1988). , 81(2), 442-8.

[29] Crowther, C. A, Hiller, J. E, Moss, J. R, et al. Effect of treatment of gestational diabetes mellitus. N Engl J Med (2005). , 352(24), 2477-86.

[30] Langer, O, Cornway, D. L, Berkus, M. D, et al. A comparison of glyburide and insulin in GDM. N Engl J Med.(2000). , 343(16), 1134-8.

[31] Anjalakshi, C, Balaji, V, Balaji, M. S, et al. A Prospective Study Comparing Insulin and Glibenclamide In Gestational Diabetes Mellitus In Asian Indian Women. Dia Res Clin Pract.(2007). , 76(3), 474-5.

[32] Glueck, C J, Wang, P, Kobayashi, S, Phillips, H, & Sieve-smith, L. Metformin therapy throughout pregnancy reduces the development of gestational diabetes in women with polycystic ovary syndrome. Fertil Steril (2002). , 77, 520-525.

[33] Begum, M. R, Khanam, N. N, Quadir, E, Ferdous, J, Begum, M. S, Khan, F, & Begum, A. Prevention of GDM by continuing metformin therapy throughout pregnancy in women with polycystic ovary syndrome (PCOS). J. Obstet. Gynaecol. (2009). , 35(2), 282-286.

[34] Glueck, C. J, Goldenberg, N, Pranikoff, J, et al. Height, weight and motor- social development during the first 18 months of life in 126 infants born to 109 mothers with polycystic ovary syndrome who conceived on and continued Metformin throughout pregnancy. Hum Reprod.(2004). , 19(6), 1323-30.

[35] Schmidt, M. I, Duncan, B. B, Reichelt, A. J, Branchtein, L, & Matos, M. C. Costa e Forti A et al for the Brazilian Gestational Diabetes Study Group. Gestational diabetes mellitus diagnosed with a 2-h 75-g oral glucose tolerance test and adverse pregnancy outcomes. Diabetes Care. (2001). , 24(7), 1151-55.

[36] Balaji, V, Madhuri, B. S, Ashalatha, S, et al. A1c in gestational diabetes mellitus in Indian Asian women. Diabetes Care, (2007). , 30(7), 1865-67.

[37] Carpenter, M. W, Canick, J. A, Hogan, J. W, Shellum, C, Somers, M, & Star, J. A. Amniotic fluid insulin at 14-20 weeks' gestation: association with later maternal glucose intolerance and birth macrosomia. Diabetes Care (2001). , 24(7), 1259-63.

[38] Bartha, J. L, Martinez-del-fresno, P, & Comino-delgado, R. Gestational diabetes mellitus diagnosed during early pregnancy, Am J Obstet Gynecol. (2000). , 182(2), 346-50.

[39] Kjos, SL, & Buchanan, . . Gestational diabetes mellitus: the prevalence of glucose intolerance and diabetes mellitus in the first two months postpartum. AM J Obstet Gynecol 1990;163:93-98.

[40] Philipson, E. H, & Super, D. N. Gestational diabetes mellitus: does it recur in subsequent pregnancy? AM J Obstet Gynecol (1989)., 160, 1324-31.

[41] Grant, P. T, Oats, J. N, & Beischer, N. The long term follow up of women with gestational diabetes. Aust N Z J Obstet Gynecol (1986).

[42] Dabelea, D, Knowler, W. C, & Pettitt, D. J. Effect of diabetes in pregnancy and offspring:follow up research in the Pima Indians. J Matern Fetal Medicine.(2000).

[43] Savona- Ventura, C, & Chircop, M. Birth weight influence on the Subsequent development of gestational diabetes mellitus. Acta Diabetol.(2003).

[44] Aerts, L. (2004). Intergenerative transmission of DM. Abstract volume of the 36th Annual Meeting of the DPSG, Luso- Portugal, September 2004.

Chapter 2

Multidisciplinary Care of Pregnant Women with Gestational Diabetes Mellitus: Non-Pharmacological Strategies to Improve Maternal and Perinatal Outcomes

Elaine Christine Dantas Moisés

Additional information is available at the end of the chapter

http://dx.doi.org/10.5772/55295

1. Introduction

Diabetes Mellitus (DM) is an endocrine disorder characterized by hyperglycemia due to insulin deficiency. This deficiency can be caused by reduced pancreatic production, inadequate release in response to increased carbohydrates or peripheral insulin resistance (ADA, 2009).

2. Classification

The first classification for Diabetes Mellitus has been published in 1949 by White Priscilla, categorizing this pathology in classes A, B, C, D, E, F, R, H and T, according to the severity of the disease, age of onset, duration, need for insulin use and the presence or absence of vascular disease arising from the Diabetes Mellitus. This classification is still widely used for predicting complications during pregnancy and is considered as an etiologic and prognostic system (Calderon et al., 2007).

The National Diabetes Data Group (1979) suggested a clinical classification based on the type of Diabetes Mellitus, considering three groups: insulin-dependent Diabetes Mellitus or Type I, Non-insulin-dependent Diabetes mellitus or Type II, and Gestational Diabetes Mellitus (GDM), which is diagnosed during pregnancy. This classification was recommended in 1980 by the World Health Organization Expert Committee on Diabetes Mellitus, being included in the same group of glucose intolerance. This classification was intended to establish a uniform structure for clinical and epidemiological research (Bennett, 1985).

The American Diabetes Association (ADA) restructured the classification and diagnostic criteria for Diabetes mellitus in 1999, emphasizing its etiology. Subsequently, the ADA (2005) ratified this classification recognized two intermediate stages of the disease, being called pre-diabetes, characterized by impaired glucose tolerance and fasting glucose intolerance (Table 1).

I. Diabetes mellitus type 1: beta-cell destruction, usually leading to absolute insulin deficiency
II. Type 2 diabetes mellitus: can vary from primarily due to insulin resistance with relative insulin deficiency to a predominantly secretory defect with insulin resistance
III. Other specific types Genetic defects of beta cell function Genetic defects in insulin action Diseases of the exocrine pancreas Endocrinopathies Drug or chemical induced Infection Unusual forms of Diabetes immunomediated Other genetic syndromes sometimes associated with diabetes IV. Gestational diabetes mellitus

Table 1. Etiological classification of Diabetes mellitus (adapted from ADA, 2005; ADA, 2009).

3. Epidemiological data on pregnancy

The dysglycemia is the most common metabolic disorder in pregnancy, but its frequency varies worldwide and among racial and ethnic groups. Broadly in general, the prevalence of dysglycemia during pregnancy can be up to 13%, corresponding to 0.1% of type 1 diabetes (T1DM), 2-3% of type 2 diabetes (T2DM) and 12 to 13% Gestational Diabetes Mellitus, depending on the diagnostic criteria used and the population studied (Hod; Diamant, 1991).

GDM is defined as glucose intolerance of variable severity, which appears or is first diagnosed during pregnancy (ADA, 2009), disappears after childbirth and that does not correspond to a pre-gestational diabetes (ADA, 2011). There has been a significant increase in the number of diagnoses of GDM over time, possibly related to an increase in average maternal weight and age (Getahun et al, 2008). Prevalence also varies according to the method of testing and diagnostic criteria.

It is recommended the early screening of high-risk pregnant women in the first prenatal visit, which allows identifying preexisting diabetes mellitus cases, which should not be erroneously termed as gestational diabetes. Excluding preexisting diabetes mellitus, pregnancy calls for the testing of employing glucose overload, from the second trimester of gestation for the diagnosis of GDM. Currently, the American Diabetes Association (ADA, 2011) and the International Association of Diabetes and Pregnancy Study Groups (IADPSG, 2010) recommend 75-g oral glucose tolerance test, with a duration of 2 hours, adopting as diagnostic criteria for GDM cutoff points suggested by the Hyperglycemia and Adverse Pregnancy Outcomes-HAPO study (2008), with plasma levels of fasting glucose greater than or equal 92 mg / dl one hour post glucose load, greater than or equal 180 mg / dl two hours post glucose load, greater than or equal 153 mg / dl, requiring only a single point change for the diagnosis of GDM. Using the diagnostic criteria proposed by IADPSG, there is detection rate of diabetes during pregnancy in about 18% of pregnant women.

4. Glycemic control

The assessment of glycemic control, through laboratory evaluation of fasting and postprandial blood glucose, supplemented with daily home blood glucose self-monitoring, should be considered every one to two weeks by the treating physician or a member of the multidisciplinary team.

Glycemic control is considered appropriate if blood glucose levels remain within the reference values (fasting less than 95 mg / dl, before meals less than 100 mg / dl, one hour postprandial less than 140 mg / dl, two hours postprandial less than 120 mg / dl) and glycosylated hemoglobin test is less than or equal to 6%. The permanence of the blood glucose above the reference values indicates the need for adjustment or inclusion of pharmacological and non-pharmacological therapies (ADA, 2011).

The criterion of excessive fetal growth, through the measurement of fetal abdominal circumference greater than or equal to the 70th percentile on ultrasound between the 29th and 33rd week, can also be used to indicate drug therapy in GDM (Buchanan et al, 1994).

5. Multidisciplinary care for pregnant women with diabetes mellitus

During prenatal care, it is essential to focus on providing information to patients about the pathophysiology and prognosis of diabetes mellitus, either pre-existing or gestational. Therefore, consultation should include targeted guidelines for diabetes care, in addition to whole routine prenatal. Its periodicity depends directly on glycemic control, beyond existence and progression of maternal and fetal complications, detected by clinical examination and complementary propaedeutic, whose discussion is not the focus of this chapter.

Poorly controlled DM is often associated with increased risks of adverse maternal and perinatal outcomes. Education and care programs in diabetes, provided by multidisciplinary team in support of the medical staff, acting either alone or associated with pharmacological treatment, may determine changes in the natural history of the disease, improving maternal and perinatal outcomes.

6. Nutritionist: Adequacy of food habit to nutritional need

Initial treatment of GDM and important part of preexisting diabetes treatment consist of nutritional guidance to provide appropriate levels of caloric intake for adequate weight gain during pregnancy, normalization of glycemia, absence of ketones and promote fetal well-being.

Dietary recommendations follow similar patterns to those aimed at the general population. The nutritional prescription constitutes the calculation of caloric intake and mounting the daily menu, in addition to providing basic concepts about nutrition, healthy eating, the food pyramid and food fractionation to the patient in order to arouse attention to the importance of nutrition in pregnancy.

The ideal weight should preferably be achieved prior to pregnancy, since that is the determining factor of the optimum setting of the nutrition prescription throughout gestation cycle. The calculation of caloric value diet and adequate weight gain can be made according to the idealized tables for this purpose (table 2), based on the Body Mass Index prior to pregnancy, frequency and intensity of physical exercises and fetal growth pattern (Kaiser, Allen, 2008).

Nutritional status	BMI prior to pregnancy (Kg/m^2)	Total weight gain in the first trimester (Kg)	Weekly weight gain in the second and third trimesters (Kg)	Total weight gain in the pregnancy (Kg)
Underweight	< 18.5	2.3	0.5	12.5 - 18
Normal Weight	18.5 – 24.9	1.6	0.4	11.5 - 16
Overweight	25.0 – 29.9	0.9	0.3	7 – 11.5
Obese	≥ 30.0	-	0.3	5 - 9

Kg: kilogram

Kg/m^2: kilograms per square meter

BMI: Body Mass Index

Table 2. Recommendation for total gain weight during pregnancy according to the Body Mass Index (BMI) before pregnancy (adapted from Kuehn, 2009).

In clinical practice, for women with BMI below 18.5 kg/m^2, the prescription of caloric intake can be up to 40 kcal / kg / day; for women with BMI between 18.5 and 24.9 kg / m^2, energy

http://dx.doi.org/10.5772/55295

intake should be 30 kcal / kg / day; for women who are overweight, the caloric supply is 22 to 25 kcal / kg / day; for the morbid obese women the caloric prescription must be from 12 to 14 kcal / kg / day.

The diet should be planned throughout the day, being split into three large meals and three snacks (ADA, 2004), being the carbohydrate intake distributed between them, aiming to prevent postprandial hyperglycemia. The nutritional requirement of carbohydrates should be restricted to less than 40% of total daily calories, with the remainder distributed among proteins (15% to 20% of total calories per day, at least 1.1 g / kg / day) and fats (30% to 40% of total calories per day). The adjustment of the postprandial insulin dose can be done by calculating the carbohydrate content of each meal.

Non-nutritive artificial sweeteners such as aspartame, saccharin, acesulfame-K and sucralose can be used sparingly, aiding the adaptation of taste to food (ADA, 2004).

7. Physical educator and therapist: Physical activity as a strategy for prevention and adjuvant treatment

Physical activity reduces insulin resistance, facilitating peripheral glucose utilization with consequent improvement of glycemic control while also helping to control weight gain during pregnancy (Reader, 2007).

The recommended exercise prescription is low-impact physical activity, ideally being practiced daily for at least 30 minutes, which can be divided into three sessions of ten minutes each, keeping levels not exceeding 50% of the aerobic capacity of the patient (table 3).

Parameter	**Programa**
Frequency	3 to 4 days / week
Intensity	Variable (according to the previous fitness)
Duration	Initially 15 minutes with gradual increase up to a maximum of 30 minutes / session
Modality	Low impact aerobic Strength training and endurance

Table 3. Prescription of exercise during pregnancy (adapted from Davies et al, 2003).

It constitutes safe method to be used during pregnancy (Szymanski, Satin, 2012). Some precautions should be observed in handling (Ferraro, Gaudet, Adamo, 2012), such as starting the physical activity sessions preferably after meals, avoiding beginning if the blood glucose is below 60 mg / dL or above 250 mg / dL (Artal, 2003). The practice of physical exercises during pregnancy is also contraindicated in cases of obstetric complications and / or concomitant medical complications, as reported in Table 4.

Obstetric contraindications	Clinical contraindications
Previous Miscarriage or preterm childbirth	Cardiovascular disease
Cervical incompetence	Hypertensive disease
Premature rupture of membranes	Respiratory disease
Preterm labor	Anemia (Hb <10 g/dl)
Intrauterine growth restriction	Malnutrition or eating disorder
Multiple pregnancy: (two fetuses after 28th week or three or more fetuses at any gestational age)	Uncontrolled Diabetes Mellitus Type 1
	Decompensated thyroid disease
Placenta previa after 28th week	
Persistent bleeding in the second and / or third trimesters	

Hb: hemoglobin

g/dl: grams per deciliter

Table 4. Contraindications to physical exercise during pregnancy (adapted from Davies et al, 2003).

8. Psychologist: Emotional support as a strategy for treatment adherence

Pregnancy, by itself, constitutes a period marked by several changes in women's lives, involving social, biological, marital and psychological changes, which are aggravated because of the occurrence of clinical and / or obstetric conditions that may potentially alter the maternal and / or fetal outcomes. These changes may act as stressors and may interfere in a positively or negatively way in adherence to the proposed treatment.

Psychological care has an evaluative component and, on the other hand, it also has an instructional feature that serves as a basis for reflection and construction of behavior in the situation experienced.

The initial characterization of the social, emotional and psychological aspects involving a pregnant woman can be accomplished through evaluation instruments (Cohen, Kamarck, Mermelstein, 1983; Zigmond, Snaith, 1983; Sherbourne, Stewart, 1991; Herrmann, 1997).

Regarding psychological intervention approach should initially focus on the demands related to pregnancy and Diabetes Mellitus brought by the patient herself and, subsequently, expand the focus to the instructional aspect, based on the information acquired. The understanding of the whole process of health care and the benefits of the proposed interventions are the basis for building the strategy of treatment adherence, particularly with regard to diet (Gardner et al, 2012).

9. Nurse: Combination of communication strategies and training techniques

Nursing staff has fundamental integrator role in the care program for pregnant women with diabetes mellitus. It features functions such as consolidation of primary communication channel created by other professionals, technical training of specialized care and monitoring of metabolic control of patient.

Different communication strategies can be adopted in order to achieve success in providing guidance and establishing appropriate relationship with patients, that allow effective training techniques of glycemic control monitoring. The establishment of this open channel of communication between the patient and nursing staff provides another opportunity to solidify concepts, in addition to allowing the sharing of anxieties and doubts, minimized by this team of professionals, collaborating to treatment adherence (Furskog et al, 2012; Mendelson et al, 2008; Persson et al, 2011).

Active and constant participation of nursing staff in the monitoring of glycemic control can determine the establishment of the patient's attention to self-care and, consequently, the drop in rates of adverse events, improving maternal-fetal prognosis (Ferrara et al, 2012)

10. Social worker: Creation of favorable environmental conditions for the treatment

The Social Services is responsible for providing guidance on social rights and social security, as well as duties related to treatment. Actions related to insertion of pregnant women in social support networks can facilitate access to certain resources, which allows better adherence to treatment and success of such proposals.

The social worker must also foster opportunities for discussion in order to create conditions for pregnant women develop their critical capacity as subjects of rights.

Reviews regarding the effectiveness of interventions offered to women during pregnancy who have been identified with social risk factors in relation to the development of depression and adherence to clinical follow-up are under development in literature (Kenyon et al, 2012).

11. Multidisciplinary group: Strategy of sharing experiences

Considering that the behavior of a pregnant woman can act as a multiplier of information and influence the conduct of another patient, it is possible to use pregnant women with adequate adhesion to treatment as a reference to be followed. In this context, multidisciplinary care with groups of diabetic pregnant women can be an effective complementary strategy to individual assistance.

Acknowledgements

To the multidisciplinary team of Clinical Hospital of Faculty of Medicine of Ribeirão Preto, University of São Paulo:

Psychologist: Juliana Caseiro

Social Worker: Renata Cecílio

Nutritionist: Daniella Cristina Fernandes da Silva

Head nurse: Ana Lúcia Moreira Fernandes

Author details

Elaine Christine Dantas Moisés

Department of Gynecology and Obstetrics, Faculty of Medicine of Ribeirão Preto, University of São Paulo, Brazil

References

[1] American Diabetes Association (2005). Diagnosis and Classification of Diabetes Mellitus. Diabetes Care28 (Suppl 1):SS42., 37.

[2] American Diabetes Association (2009). Diagnosis and Classification of Diabetes Mellitus. Diabetes Care 32 (Suppl 1): SS67., 62.

[3] American Diabetes Association- ReportsPosition of the American Dietetic Association: use of nutritive and nonnutritive sweeteners (2004). J Am Diet Assoc., 255-275.

[4] American Diabetes Association (2011). Standards of medical care in diabetes-2011. Diabetes Care 34 (Suppl 1): SS61., 11.

[5] Artal, R. (2003). Exercise: the alternative therapeutic intervention for gestational diabetes. Clin Obstet Gynecol, 46(2), 479-487.

[6] Bennett, P. H. (1985). Basis of the present classification of Diabetes. Adv Exp Med Biol., 189, 17-29.

[7] Buchanan, T, Kjos, S. L, & Montoro, M. N. Wu PYK, Madrilejo NG, Gonzales M (1994). Use of fetal ultrasound to select metabolic therapy for pregnancies complicated by mild diabetes. Diabetes Care, 17, 275-283.

[8] Calderon IMPKerche LTRL, Damasceno DC, Rudge MVC (2007). Diabetes and Pregnancy: an Update of the Problem. ARBS Annu Rev Biomed Sci, 9, 1-11.

[9] Cohen, S, Kamarck, T, & Mermelstein, R. (1983). A global measure of perceived stress. J Health Soc Behav, 24(4), 385-396.

[10] Davies, G. A, Wolfe, L. A, & Mottola, M. F. MacKinnon C; Society of Obstetricians and gynecologists of Canada, SOGC Clinical Practice Obstetrics Committee (2003). Joint SOGC/CSEP clinical practice guideline: exercise in pregnancy and the postpartum period. Can J Appl Physiol, 28(3), 330-341.

[11] Ferrara, A, Hedderson, M. M, Ching, J, Kim, C, Peng, T, & Crites, Y. M. (2012). Referral to telephonic nurse management improves outcomes in women with gestational diabetes. Am J Obstet Gynecol206(6):491.e, 1-5.

[12] Ferraro, Z. M, Gaudet, L, & Adamo, K. B. (2012). The potential impact of physical activity during pregnancy on maternal and neonatal outcomes.Obstet Gynecol Surv, 67(2), 99-110.

[13] Furskog Risa C, Friberg F, Lidén E (2012). Experts' encounters in antenatal diabetes care: a descriptive study of verbal communication in midwife-led consultations. Nurs Res Pract2012:121360

[14] Gardner, B, Croker, H, Barr, S, Briley, A, Poston, L, & Wardle, J. UPBEAT Trial (2012). Psychological predictors of dietary intentions in pregnancy. J Hum Nutr Diet , 25(4), 345-353.

[15] Getahun, D, Nath, C, Ananth, C. V, Chavez, M. R, & Smulian, J. C. (2008). Gestational diabetes in the United States: temporal trends 1989 through 2004. Am J Obstet Gynecol 198(5):525.e, 1-5.

[16] HAPO Study Cooperative Research GroupMetzger BE, Lowe LP, Dyer AR, Trimble ER, Chaovarindr U, Coustan DR, Hadden DR, McCance DR, Hod M, McIntyre HD, Oats JJ, Persson B, Rogers MS, Sacks DA ((2008). Hyperglycemia and adverse pregnancy outcomes. N Engl J Med , 358(19), 1991-2002.

[17] Herrmann, C. (1997). International experiences with the Hospital Anxiety and Depression Scale--a review of validation data and clinical results. J Psychosom Res, 42(1), 17-41.

[18] Hod, M, & Diamant, Y. Z. (1991). Diabetes in pregnancy. Norbert Freinkel Memorial Issue. Isr J Med Sci, 27, 421-532.

[19] International Association of Diabetes and Pregnancy Study Groups Consensus Panel-Metzger BE, Gabbe SG, Persson B, Buchanan TA, Catalano PA, Damm P, Dyer AR, Leiva A, Hod M, Kitzmiler JL, Lowe LP, McIntyre HD, Oats JJ, Omori Y, Schmidt MI

((2010). International association of diabetes and pregnancy study groups recommendations on the diagnosis and classification of hyperglycemia in pregnancy. Diabetes Care, 33(3), 676-682.

[20] Kaiser, L, & Allen, L. H. (2008). Position of the American Dietetic Association: nutrition and lifestyle for a healthy pregnancy outcome. J Am Diet Assoc, 108(3), 553-561.

[21] Kenyon, S, Jolly, K, Hemming, K, Ingram, L, Gale, N, Dann, S. A, & Chambers, J. MacArthur C (2012). Evaluation of Lay Support in Pregnant women with Social risk (ELSIPS): a randomised controlled trial. BMC Pregnancy Childbirth12:11.

[22] Kuehn, B. M. (2009). Guideline for pregnancy weight gain offers targets for obese women. JAMA, 302(3), 241-242.

[23] Mendelson, S. G, Mcneese-smith, D, Koniak-griffin, D, Nyamathi, A, & Lu, M. C. parish nurse intervention program for Mexican American women with gestational diabetes. J Obstet Gynecol Neonatal Nurs, 37(4), 415-425.

[24] National Academy of Sciences Institute of Medicine, Food and Nutrition Board, Committee on Nutritional Status During Pregnancy and Lactation, Subcommittee for a Clinical Application Guide: Nutrition During Pregnancy and Lactation: An Implementation Guide. Washington, D.C., National Academies Press (1992).

[25] Persson, M, Hörnsten, A, Winkvist, A, & Mogren, I. (2011). Mission impossible"? Midwives' experiences counseling pregnant women with gestational diabetes mellitus. Patient Educ Couns, 84(1), 78-83.

[26] Sherbourne, C. D, & Stewart, A. L. (1991). The MOS social support survey. Soc Sci Med, 32(6), 705-14.

[27] Szymanski, L. M, & Satin, A. J. (2012). Exercise during pregnancy: fetal responses to current public health guidelines. Obstet Gynecol, 119(3), 603-10.

[28] Zigmond, A. S, & Snaith, R. P. (1983). The hospital anxiety and depression scale. Acta Psychiatr Scand, 67(6), 361-70.

Section 2

Cell and Molecular Mechanisms

Chapter 3

The Role of Placental Exosomes in Gestational Diabetes Mellitus

Carlos Salomon, Luis Sobrevia, Keith Ashman, Sebastian E. Illanes, Murray D. Mitchell and Gregory E. Rice

Additional information is available at the end of the chapter

http://dx.doi.org/10.5772/55298

1. Introduction

Gestational Diabetes Mellitus (GDM) affects ~5% of all pregnancies and parallels the global increase in obesity and type 2 diabetes. In the USA alone, GDM affects more than 135,000 pregnancies per year. Lifestyle changes that impact adversely on caloric balance are thought to be a contributing factor in this emerging pandemic [1, 2]. The current 'gold standard' for the diagnosis of GDM is the oral glucose tolerance test (OGTT) at 24–28 weeks of gestation [3, 4]. When GDM is diagnosed in the late second or early third trimester of pregnancy the 'pathology' is most likely well-established and the possibility to reverse or limit potential adverse effects on perinatal outcomes may be limited [5]. Early detection of predisposition to and/or onset of GDM, thus, is the first step in developing, evaluating and implementing efficacious treatment. If such early detection tests were available, they would represent a major advance and contribution to the discipline and afford the opportunity to evaluate alternate treatment and clinical management strategies to improve health outcomes for both mother and baby. Based upon recent technological developments and studies, we consider it realistic that a clinically useful antenatal screening test can be developed. Unlike diseases such as cancer where biomarkers need to be exquisitely specific, a useful antenatal screening test would ideally be highly sensitive, but not necessarily highly specific. The consequence of a false positive would be no worse than an erroneous triage to high-risk care.

Recent studies highlight the putative utility of tissue-specific nanovesicles (*e.g.* exosomes) in the diagnosis of disease onset and treatment monitoring [6-11]. To date there is a paucity of data defining changes in the release, role and diagnostic utility of placenta-derived nanovesicles (*e.g.* exosomes) in pregnancies complicated by GDM.

The aim of this brief commentary, thus, is to review the biogenesis, isolation and role of nanovesicles; and their release from the placenta. Placental exosomes may engage in paracellular interactions (*i.e.* local cell-to-cell communication between the cell constituents of the placenta and contiguous maternal tissues) and/or distal interactions (*i.e.* involving the release of placental exosomes into biological fluids and their transport to a remote site of action).

2. Exosome biogenesis and composition

2.1. Biogenesis

Exosomes are small [40-100 nm) membrane vesicles that are released following the exocytotic fusion of multi-vesicular bodies with the cell membrane (Figure 1). They are characterised by: a cup-shaped form: (a) a buoyant density of 1.13-1.19 g/ml [12, 13], (b) endosomal origin, and (c) the enrichment of late endosomal membrane markers including Tsg101, CD63, CD9 and CD81 [7, 14, 15]. While the process(es) of exosome formation remains to be fully elucidated, available data support an endosomal origin and formation by the inward budding of multi-vesicular bodies [16] (see Figure 2). Exosomes may also be directly transported from the Golgi complex to multi-vesicular bodies [14].

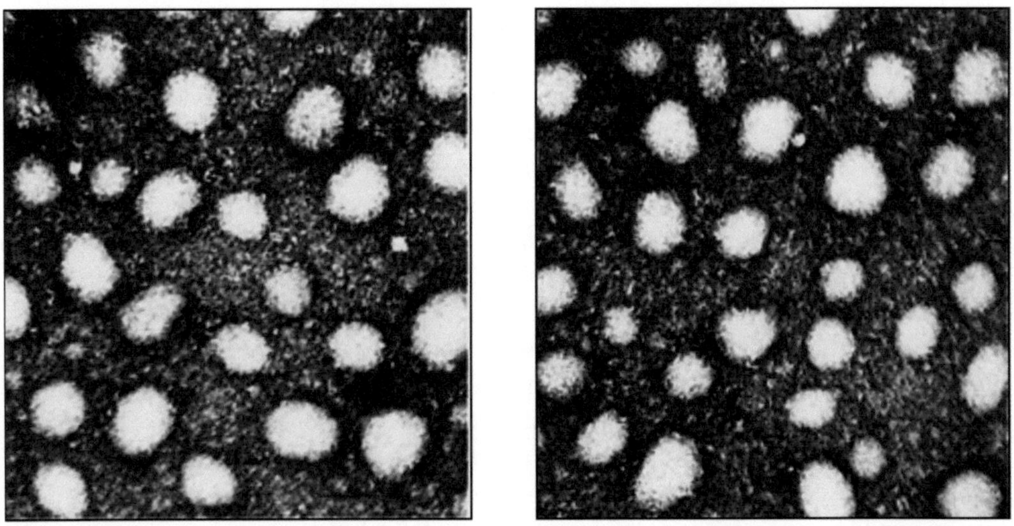

Figure 1. Electron micrograph of circulating exosomes. Exosomes are 40-100 nm membrane vesicles with a density ranging from 1.13-1.19 g/ml, characterised by a cup-shaped form and secreted by most cell types *in vivo* and *in vitro*. Villous chorionic explant-derived exosomes were isolated by ultracentrifugation and purified using a sucrose gradient. Scale bar = 100 nm.

http://dx.doi.org/10.5772/55298

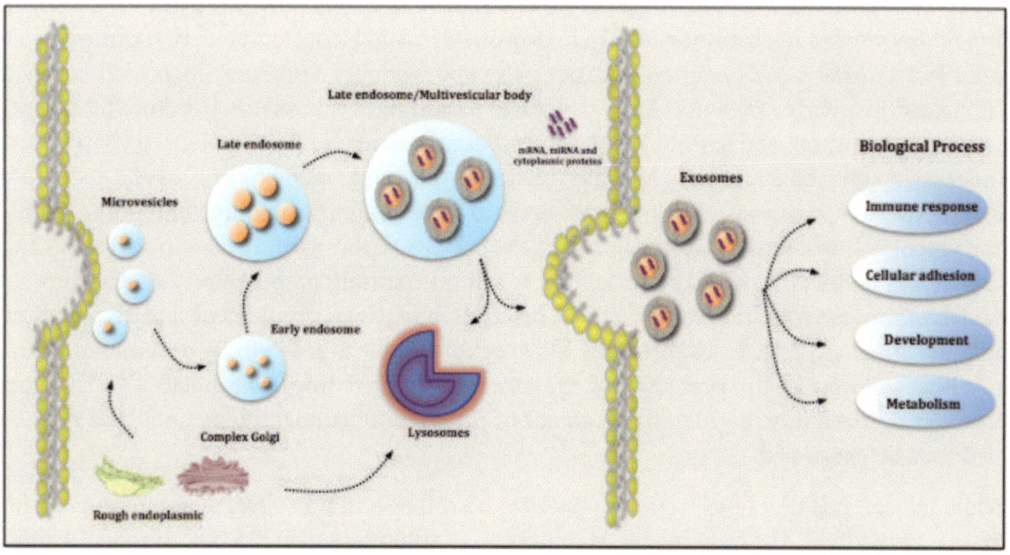

Figure 2. Schematic of exosome biogenesis and secretion. Exosomes are generated in the endosomal structure participating the plasma membrane in this process, and secreted via constitutive endosomal pathways involving the Golgi complex from various cell types. The exosomes contain specific proteins and miRNA as a new form of exosome-mediated intercellular communication and with different biological function. In pathological pregnancies characterised by compromised placental perfusion and ischaemia, such as GDM, exosome secreted from the placenta can participate in an adaptive response of the mother and fetus and so interact with target tissue and modulate different biological processes, such as immune response, cellular adhesion, development and metabolism.

Exosomes have been identified in plasma under both normal and pathological conditions. The concentration of exosomal protein in plasma has been reported to increase in association with disease severity and/or progression, and in response to oxidative stress. Cell membrane budding and the deportation of cell membrane particles was originally considered as the elimination of cell debris and associated with apoptosis and/or necrosis. Recent data, however, suggest that the release of nanovesicles from cells may represent a normal mechanism for cell-to-cell communication [17]. Packaging of exosomal contents appears to be a direct process in which the ESCRT (endosomal sorting complex required for transport) systems play a significant role [18-20].

Exosomes are released from the placenta and the concentration of exosomes in maternal plasma increases during normal pregnancy [21-23]. *In vitro*, exosomes are released from both trophoblast cells and syncytium [24]. They contain placenta-specific proteins and miRNA and, as such, may be differentiated from maternally-derived exosomes [25]. The concentration of exosomes has been reported to increase in association with pre-eclampsia [22, 23, 26]. The role of exosomes in the development and progression of GDM has yet to be established.

2.2. Composition

The exosomal content is highly dependent on the origin cell and on pre-conditioning of the cell. One of the first exosomal proteomes characterised was from mesothelioma cells, in which

38 different proteins were identified [27]. Studies in cancer cells show the great variability of proteins expressed in exosomes [28-32]. In exosomes isolated from a human first trimester cell line (Sw7 1) Atay *et al.,* using an ion trap mass spectrometry approach, identified proteins implicated in a wide range of cellular processes including: cytoskeleton structure (adhesion, membrane transport, and fusion), ion channels, lysosomal degradation, molecular chaperones, amino-acid metabolism, carbohydrate metabolism, lipid metabolism, oxydo-reductase activity, protein synthesis and post-translational modifications, ubiquitin modifiers, signal transduction, transcription factors and regulators, DNA replication, chromatin structural and regulatory proteins, mRNA splicing, transcription/translation, post-translational protein modification enzymes, nuclear structural proteins, integrins, complement and coagulation, immune function, iron transport, and ER specific proteins. This study provides the first extensive analysis of the proteome of the exosome-derived trophoblast cells [7]. The data obtained in this study, highlights the extent of putative functional interactions that may be mediated by exosomes.

While the composition of exosomes appears to be cell-specific, a subset of common proteins has been identified. The lipid bilayer is composed of sphingomyelin [33, 34]. Among the most commonly used markers for characterisation of exosomes are tetraspanin proteins, including: CD63, CD81, CD9, and CD82. Other families of common proteins in all exosomes include chaperone proteins such as: Hsc70 and Hsp90; cytoskeletal proteins including actin, tubulin and myosin; transport proteins; and annexins [35]. Exosomes derived from antigen-presenting cells (APC) express MHC-I and MHC-II on their surface [36-38]. During exosome biogenesis, the phospholipid/protein ratio of exosomes may be regulated by the Golgi membranes [39].

Significantly, single cell types display the capacity to generate different subpopulations of exosomes. Laulagnier *et al.* 2005 demonstrated that RBL-2H3 cells (basophilic leukemia cell line) released two main subpopulations of exosomes that can be discriminated by protein and lipid contents. The first subpopulation contains phospholipids obtained mainly from granules and the second contains phospholipids from Golgi. In addition, proteins CD63, MHC-II, CD81-containing exosomes accounted for 47%, 32%, and 21%, respectively, of total exosomes [39, 40].

3. Isolation of exosomes

Exosome research is a burgeoning discipline with over 2000 articles published in the last 3 years. The putative role of exosomes spans from intracellular signaling to biomarkers of disease [41]. Germane to any study seeking to elucidate the physiological or pathophysiological role of exosomes is their specific isolation. Several methods for isolating exosomes have been developed and partially characterised. These isolation methods are primarily based on particle size and density. By definition, exosomes are nanovesicles with a diameter of 30-100 nm. Typically they display a density of 1.12 to 1.19 g/ml and express characteristic cell-surface markers.

The most common method of separation involves a series of differential centrifugation to remove intact cells and debris, and nuclei followed by size selective filtration (0.2 μm pore size) and sedimentation by ultracentrifugation (*e.g.* at 110,000 g for 1-2 hours [42, 43]. Exosomes may be further purified by differential sedimentation on sucrose gradients or sucrose-deuterium oxide (D_2O) [7]. Alternative methods utilise size exclusion chromatography and density gradient centrifugation [44] or solid-phase immunoaffinity capture (*i.e.* anti-MHC-II Dynabeads) [38, 43, 45]. In the absence of specific, cell surface exosome markers, the veracity of immuno-affinity methods remains to be established.

More recently a commercial kit for the isolation of the exosomes has been released (ExoQuick™, System Biosciences). The isolation process involves a simple one-step precipitation [43, 46]. While the commercial kit provides significant advantage with respect to processing time, the resulting preparation may not be equivalent to that obtained by ultracentrifugation and differential segmentation. In our own laboratory, parallel preparations of exosomes using both methods reveal differences in the biophysical characteristics of the exosomes isolated. Exosome preparations isolated using the commercial kit were characterised by a great range in particle diameter (30-300 nm, as estimated by transmission electron microscopy (TEM) and have a higher protein content than similar preparations isolated using the ultracentrifugation method. In addition, analysis of protein patterns in SDS-PAGE electrophoresis and western blot against CD63, CD81 and CD9 show similar characteristics between exosomes from ultracentrifuge and ExoQuick™ methods, however, we had to dilute ExoQuick™ samples ~ 10 times to obtain comparable concentrations with ultracentrifuge methods in exosomes isolated from trophoblastic cells (see Figure 3). Differences in exosome protein and mRNA content and functional activity between different preparations remain to be established.

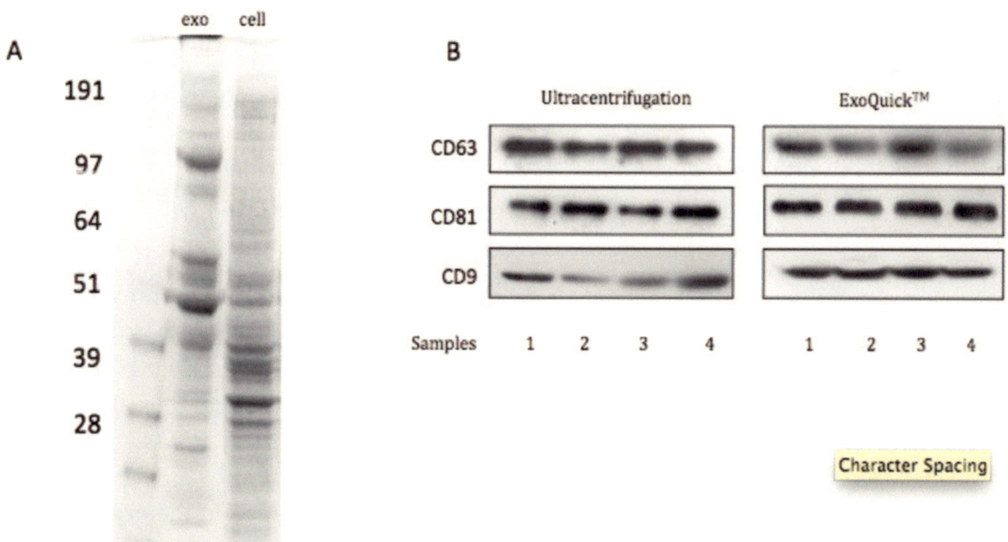

Figure 3. Typical characteristics of exosomes isolated from trophoblast cells. (A) Exosome protein pattern analysis. 10 ug of exosome proteins and trophoblast cell lysate were separated on 4-12% SDS-PAGE and stained with SimplyBlue™ SafeStain (Invitrogen). (B) Western blot characterisation of exosomes with antibodies against CD63, CD81 and CD9 for 4 different samples isolated with ultracentrifuge or ExoQuick™ methods.

4. The role for exosomes in cell-to-cell communication

Recently, evidence supporting a role for exosomes in cell-to-cell communication has been obtained [47, 48]. Exosome release may represent a significant, hitherto unappreciated, communication mechanism between cells, host cell and microbes [47].

For example, exosome function as a carrier of specific molecules such as mRNA and miRNA can interact with neighbouring cells or travel long distances in the bloodstream to reprogram the phenotype and regulate their function [40]. In the placenta, exosome- derived trophoblastic cells are able to reprogram monocytes to secrete specific cytokine profiles independent of cell-to-cell contact [8]. Placental-derived exosomes may also play a role in modulating immunological responses through the induction of lymphocyte apoptosis, [21, 44, 49].

4.1. Information encoding by exosomes

Exosomes have been reported to express a diverse range of cell surface receptors, proteins (including, heat shock proteins, cytoskeletal proteins, adhesion molecules, membrane transport and fusion proteins), mRNA and miRNA with the potential to affect the acute and long-term function of the cells with which they interact [50]. In addition, in the absence of energy production, normal membrane phospholipid asymmetry is lost and amniophospholipids translocate to the outer leaflet of the cell membrane and generate a fusogenic and pro-coagulant surface. Given that exosomes circulate in blood, these fusogenic moieties may be masked by, for example, annexin V.

In vitro effects of exposing cells to exosomal proteins has been reported and include: induction of differentiation of stem cells [51], suppression of activation of natural killer cells and macrophages [52, 53], and stimulation of cell migration [8, 54]. Putative roles of exosomes, thus, include cell differentiation, immunomodulation and migration [55]. Exosomes are not merely inert fragments of cell membrane but display capacity to affect cell function at remote loci and possibly be a source of disease biomarkers.

Exosomes also contain miRNA that may transfer to other cells and alter the expression of the transcriptome and ultimately cell phenotype. miRNAs are a class of small non-coding RNAs that function as translational repressors involved in a variety of physiological and pathological processes in animals [56, 57]. They act via binding to messenger RNA and, thus, prevent the translation of the encoded protein. Previous studies have reported that miRNAs are involved in the pathogenesis of diabetes and are required for pancreatic development and the regulation of glucose-stimulated insulin secretion [50, 58]. Moreover, differences in the expression of miRNA such as miR-146a, miR-21, miR-29a, miR-34a, miR-222, and miR-375 have been reported in pancreatic β-cells, liver, adipose tissue, and/or skeletal muscle of animal models of type 1 or type 2 diabetes [59]. Another study found that miR-20b, miR-21, miR-24, miR-15a, miR-126, miR-191, miR-197, miR-223, miR-320, and miR-486 were lower in prevalent type 2 diabetes [60].

4.2. Placental exosome release and effects

4.2.1. Placental exosome release

Exosomes are released by the placenta during pregnancy and their release may correlate with pregnancy outcome. The syncytiotrophoblasts and cytotrophoblasts are the most abundant cell types of the human placenta and sense and regulate oxygen and nutritional exchange between mother and fetus during the pregnancy [61, 62]. Pathologies of pregnancy including preeclampsia, intrauterine growth restriction (IUGR) and GDM are associated with placental dysfunction [4, 63, 64] and may display differential and specific exosome release profiles.

It has been established that the concentration of exosomes in maternal peripheral blood is greater than that observed in non-pregnant women [21]. In this study, exosomes of placental origin were specifically isolated from the maternal blood using anti-PLAP (anti-placental-type alkaline phosphatase) conjugated to agarose micro-beads. In peripheral blood mononuclear cells (PBMC), placental exosomes suppressed T signalling components such as CD3-zeta and JAK3, while inducing SOCS-2 [2 1]. These results are consistent with those of Taylor *et al.* [44, 65] who demonstrated the presence and composition of placenta-derived exosomes in maternal circulation along with their effects on T cell activation markers. Exosomes appear to play an essential role in preventing an excessive immune response and in the development of autoimmunity in human pregnancy.

Recently, it has been demonstrated that placental miRNAs circulate in the blood of pregnant women [66, 67]. For example, maternal plasma concentration of placental miRNA-141 increases with gestational age [66]. Placenta-specific miRNA-517A is released from chorionic villous trophoblasts into maternal circulation, where it may affect maternal tissues (*e.g.* maternal endothelium) during pregnancy [25]. There is a paucity of data, however characterising the release of exosome from endothelial cells during normal and pathological pregnancies. It will be important to determine if the placenta communicates with the maternal endothelium via microvesicles, and, if so, to elucidate the role and mechanism of action of exosome pathologies associated with endothelial dysfunction, such as GDM. Placenta-derived miRNAs, therefore, may be of utility as biomarkers of placental function and/or pregnancy outcome. It remains to be elucidated how much of this "free" miRNA and mRNA is actually contained within exosomes and thereby confers stability. Indeed, the exact mechanisms involved in the release of miRNA from the placenta remain to be established. A recent study, however, reported that miRNAs are selectively packaged into microvesicles and are actively secreted [68-70]. miRNAs are also released from the syncytiotrophoblast to the maternal circulation in the pregnancy packaged inside exosomes [25, 71].

4.2.2. Effects

There remains a paucity of data about the effect of placenta-derived exosomes on both fetus and mother. The available data, however, support a role for placental exosomes in mediating communication at the materno-fetal interface and, possibly, at the distal site within the mother. Recent data show that trophoblast-derived exosomes induce proinflammatory cytokines such IL-1 β in human macrophages cells [8]. Furthermore, *in vitro* exposure of PBMC and dendritic cells to exosomal proteins induce differentiation of stem cells; suppression of activation of natural killer cells and macrophages; and stimulation of cell migration [53, 72, 73]. Interestingly, protein analysis revealed that exosome release from trophoblast cells increases with low oxygen tension and their exosome promote the cell migration in extravillous cytotrophoblast (HTR- 8) (Salomon et al. manuscript in preparation).

5. Exosomes and GDM

Exosomes released from the placentae of women with GDM may alter maternal physiology. Via a process of *exosomal placento-maternal transfection* a "payload" of receptors, proteins and/or oligonucleotides" that have been specifically pre-conditioned by the GDM placenta may be delivered to maternal response systems. Such mediators include: vascular, pancreatic and adipose tissues, and the innate immune response system. The extent and impact of placenta-derived exosomes on maternal physiology, however, remains to be elucidated.

In addition to a *placento-maternal transfection* pathway, trophoblasts or placental mesenchymal stem cells (MSCs) may induce paracellular effects in association with GDM. For example, in placental villi, exosomes released by perivascular MSCs may alter transport activity within the placental vascular endothelium (*e.g.* the glucose transport GLUT 3) and thus the delivery of energy substrates to the fetus.

In support of the role of exosomes in modulating glucose homeostasis, Deng *et al.*, reported that exosomes isolated from adipose tissue induce differentiation of monocytes into activated macrophages and promote insulin resistance in an obese mouse model [74]. Exosomes isolated from mouse insulinoma induce the secretion of inflammatory cytokines including IL-6 and TNF-α in splenocytes cultured from non-obese diabetic mice (NOD) [75]. In this regards, these cytokines as well as other inflammatory mediators play an important role in glucose tolerance and insulin sensitivity dysregulation in women with previous GDM.

5.1. The effects of hyperglycaemia and oxidative stress on exosome release

GDM is a state of hyperglycaemia and increased oxidative stress [76]. In addition, hyperglycaemia-induced oxidative stress makes an important contribution to the aetiology of GDM [77], with consequences for both mother and baby [78]. In support of an aetiological role of hypoglycaemia and attendant oxidative stress in poor pregnancy outcome, the HAPO study reported a strong and continuous association between maternal glucose concentrations and pregnancy outcome and confirmed a relationship between birth weight and maternal hyperglycaemia [79, 80].

Reactive oxygen species (ROS) include oxygen ions such as superoxide ions and hydrogen peroxide (H_2O_2) that are generated continuously during cellular metabolism. GDM pregnancies are characterised by an overproduction of ROS and free radicals and impaired antioxidant capacity [81]. Oxidative stress and increased exosome release are common features of many pathologies including: cancer, kidney disease, hypertension, and preeclampsia. It remains to be established whether or not exosome release in these circumstances is a paraphenomenon of, or an adaptive response to, increased ROS formation and oxidative stress.

GDM is a syndrome that leads to feto-placental vascular endothelial dysfunction involving higher nitric oxide (NO) concentrations and increases of oxidative state and vascular resistance [63, 82]. Exosomes – endothelial cell interactions may result in activation of NO synthesis via a number of mechanisms. Exosomes isolated from platelets obtained from patients with septic induced endothelial dysfunction through the NADPH oxidase-dependent release of superoxide and have been implicated in the induction of NO and peroxinitrite. NO synthase is also induced by miR-203. miRNA-203 has been identified in exosomes [83]. It remains to be established whether or not miRNA-203 is present in exosomes isolated from women with GDM.

In non-gestational tissues, the available evidence supports an active role for exosomes in regulating cellular redox status. For example, oxidative stress enhances exosome release from Jurkat and Raji cell lines and the resultant increase in NKG2D receptor bioactivity impairs cytotoxic response [84]. In 3T3-L1 adipocytes, oxidative stress increases microvesicle release [85]. Melanoma-derived exosomes induce ROS production in T cells compared to exosomes from normal cells, suppressing the immune response and improving carcinogenic invasion [86]. Exosomes isolated from mouse mast cells MC/9 exposed to oxidative stress alter the response of others cells to oxidative stress [87], increasing their resistance to oxidative stress and reducing cell death. Interestingly, the mRNA content of exosomes produced under oxidative stress conditions differ from those produced under normal conditions. These data are consistent with the observations of Atay *et al.* [7, 8], Luo *et al.*, [25] and Taylor *et al.* [83] who similarly report cell- and condition-specific variation in exosomal protein, mRNA and miRNA content.

5.2. Exosome biomarkers of GDM

In addition to their putative functional involvement in the pathophysiology of pregnancy, placental-derived exosomes may be of utility as diagnostic markers of GDM in asymptomatic women.

In 2011, the American Diabetes Association (ADA) and the International Association of Diabetes and Pregnancy Study Groups (IADPSG) revised recommendations regarding GDM. It is now recommended that patients at increased risk for type 2 diabetes be screened for diabetes using standard diagnostic criteria at their first prenatal visit (ADA 201 2). Currently, GDM is diagnosed in the late second or early third trimester of pregnancy. Pathology is probably already established by this time and reversal of the potential adverse perinatal outcomes may be limited. The lack of a reliable early test for GDM has hampered the development of useful intervention therapies that may impact not only on the acute but also the long-term health outcomes [88-90]. Thus, there is a need to diagnose and predict GDM earlier so that appropriate management can be initiated and tailored to the needs of the patient in order to minimise perinatal complications and their sequelae.

Currently, the diagnosis of GDM is between 24-28 weeks of gestation by an oral glucose tolerance test. The aim of the treatment for GDM is to maintain the glucose level in euglycaemia with dietary modifications or in some cases with insulin therapy, however, when it is diagnosed, the pathology is established and the clinical and obstetric management is limited [5, 91].

The quantitation of exosomes and/or exosome-specific content may be of diagnostic utility [14, 43, 83, 92, 93]. Exosomes are found in all body fluids tested to date including blood, urine, saliva and breast milk. They can be obtained by minimally invasive methods (blood) or noninvasive methods (using urine or saliva) [94]. Several studies have demonstrated the putative utility of exosomes as biomarkers, particularly in cancers, where exosomal protein is correlated with disease burden.

The measurement of exosomal miRNA in biofluids has proven of utility in cases of lung cancer, colorectal cancer, prostate cancer and diabetes [95-99].

Zhao *et al.* isolated miRNA from blood circulation at 16-19 gestational weeks. Interestingly, these authors found that the expression of miRNA-132, miRNA-29a and miRNA-22 were decreased in GDM women compared with normal pregnancies in similar gestational weeks [70]. Finally, there are few reports suggesting that mesenchymal stem cell and trophoblast cells-derived exosomes may serve as therapeutic agents for use in regenerative medicine to repair damaged tissue [100, 101].

Finally, in normal pregnancies, the placenta secretes significant amounts of macro- and microvesicles, including exosomes [22, 26]. We suggest that in pregnancies complicated by GDM, oxidative stress and hyperglycaemia increase the release of exosomes from the placenta into the maternal circulation during in the first trimester of pregnancy. The quantification and characterised of exosomes in the blood of these pre-symptomatic women, thus, may be of utility as an early biomarker of disease onset. Furthermore, we propose that during first trimester, pre-symptomatic women who subsequently develop GDM: have higher plasma concentrations of placental-derived exosomes; and a different exosomal protein and miRNA profile than women who experience a normoglycaemic pregnancy. These characteristics could potentially be used for diagnostic markers for exosome profiling to screen asymptomatic populations.

Acknowledgements

CS holds a Postdoctoral Fellowship at The University of Queensland Centre for Clinical Research, Brisbane, Australia. GER was in receipt of an NHMRC Principal Research Fellowship. The work described herein was partially funded by a CIEF grant (University of Queensland), a Smart Futures Fund grant (Department of Employment, Economic Development and Innovation, Queensland Government) and a Translating Health Discovery into Clinical Applications SuperScience Award (Department of Industry, Innovation, Science, Research and Tertiary Education, Australian Government).

This investigation was supported by CONICYT (ACT-73 PIA, Pasantía Doctoral en el Extranjero BECAS Chile), FONDECYT (1110977). CS hold CONICYT-PhD fellowships and Faculty of Medicine/PUC-PhD fellowships.

Author details

Carlos Salomon[1,2], Luis Sobrevia[1], Keith Ashman[2], Sebastian E. Illanes[3], Murray D. Mitchell[2] and Gregory E. Rice[2]

1 Cellular and Molecular Physiology Laboratory (CMPL), Division of Obstetrics and Gynaecology, School of Medicine, Faculty of Medicine, Pontificia Universidad Católica de Chile, Santiago, Chile

2 University of Queensland Centre for Clinical Research, University of Queensland, Herston, Queensland, Australia

3 Department of Obstetric and Gynaecology, Universidad de los Andes, Santiago, Chile

References

[1] Ferrara A, Kahn HS, Quesenberry CP, Riley C, Hedderson MM. An increase in the incidence of gestational diabetes mellitus: Northern California, 1991-2000. Obstetrics and gynecology. 2004;103 (3):526-33. Epub 2004/03/03.

[2] Robitaille J, Grant AM. The genetics of gestational diabetes mellitus: evidence for relationship with type 2 diabetes mellitus. Genetics in medicine : official journal of the American College of Medical Genetics. 2008;10 (4):240-50. Epub 2008/04/17.

[3] Diagnosis and classification of diabetes mellitus. Diabetes care. 2012;35 Suppl 1:S64-71. Epub 2012/01/04.

[4] Salomon C, Westermeier F, Puebla C, Arroyo P, Guzman-Gutierrez E, Pardo F, et al. Gestational diabetes reduces adenosine transport in human placental microvascular endothelium, an effect reversed by insulin. PloS one. 2012;7 (7):e40578. Epub 2012/07/19.

[5] Agarwal MM, Weigl B, Hod M. Gestational diabetes screening: the low-cost algorithm. International journal of gynaecology and obstetrics: the official organ of the International Federation of Gynaecology and Obstetrics. 2011;115 Suppl 1:S30-3. Epub 2011/12/07.

[6] Chen Y, Ge W, Xu L, Qu C, Zhu M, Zhang W, et al. miR-200b is involved in intestinal fibrosis of Crohn's disease. International journal of molecular medicine. 2012;29 (4): 601-6. Epub 2012/02/02.

[7] Atay S, Gercel-Taylor C, Kesimer M, Taylor DD. Morphologic and proteomic characterization of exosomes released by cultured extravillous trophoblast cells. Experimental cell research. 2011;317 (8):1192-202. Epub 2011/02/01.

[8] Atay S, Gercel-Taylor C, Suttles J, Mor G, Taylor DD. Trophoblast-derived exosomes mediate monocyte recruitment and differentiation. Am J Reprod Immunol. 2011;65 (1):65-77. Epub 2010/06/22.

[9] Armitage JA, Poston L, Taylor PD. Developmental origins of obesity and the metabolic syndrome: the role of maternal obesity. Frontiers of hormone research. 2008;36:73-84. Epub 2008/01/31.

[10] Taylor DD, Gercel-Taylor C. Tumour-derived exosomes and their role in cancer-associated T-cell signalling defects. British journal of cancer. 2005;92 (2):305-11. Epub 2005/01/19.

[11] Simpson RJ, Jensen SS, Lim JW. Proteomic profiling of exosomes: current perspectives. Proteomics. 2008;8 (1 9):4083-99. Epub 2008/09/10.

[12] Mignot G, Roux S, Thery C, Segura E, Zitvogel L. Prospects for exosomes in immunotherapy of cancer. Journal of cellular and molecular medicine. 2006;10 (2):376-88. Epub 2006/06/27.

[13] Miranda KC, Bond DT, McKee M, Skog J, Paunescu TG, Da Silva N, et al. Nucleic acids within urinary exosomes/microvesicles are potential biomarkers for renal disease. Kidney international. 2010;78 (2):191-9. Epub 2010/04/30.

[14] Mincheva-Nilsson L, Baranov V. The role of placental exosomes in reproduction. Am J Reprod Immunol. 2010;63 (6):520-33. Epub 2010/03/25.

[15] Keller S, Ridinger J, Rupp AK, Janssen JW, Altevogt P. Body fluid derived exosomes as a novel template for clinical diagnostics. Journal of translational medicine. 2011;9:86. Epub 2011/06/10.

[16] Simons M, Raposo G. Exosomes--vesicular carriers for intercellular communication. Current opinion in cell biology. 2009;21 (4):575-81. Epub 2009/05/16.

[17] Ludwig AK, Giebel B. Exosomes: small vesicles participating in intercellular communication. The international journal of biochemistry & cell biology. 2012;44 (1):11-5. Epub 2011/10/26.

[18] Wegner CS, Rodahl LM, Stenmark H. ESCRT proteins and cell signalling. Traffic. 2011;12 (1 0):1291-7. Epub 2011/04/27.

[19] Stuffers S, Sem Wegner C, Stenmark H, Brech A. Multivesicular endosome biogenesis in the absence of ESCRTs. Traffic. 2009;10 (7):925-37. Epub 2009/06/06.

[20] Stuffers S, Brech A, Stenmark H. ESCRT proteins in physiology and disease. Experimental cell research. 2009;315 (9):1619-26. Epub 2008/11/18.

[21] Sabapatha A, Gercel-Taylor C, Taylor DD. Specific isolation of placenta-derived exosomes from the circulation of pregnant women and their immunoregulatory consequences. Am J Reprod Immunol. 2006;56 (5- 6):345-55. Epub 2006/11/02.

[22] Redman CW, Sargent IL. Circulating microparticles in normal pregnancy and pre-eclampsia. Placenta. 2008;29 Suppl A:S73-7. Epub 2008/01/15.

[23] Orozco AF, Lewis DE. Flow cytometric analysis of circulating microparticles in plasma. Cytometry Part A : the journal of the International Society for Analytical Cytology. 2010;77 (6):502-14. Epub 2010/03/18.

[24] Atay S, Gercel-Taylor C, Taylor DD. Human trophoblast-derived exosomal fibronectin induces pro-inflammatory IL-1beta production by macrophages. Am J Reprod Immunol. 2011;66 (4):259-69. Epub 2011/03/18.

[25] Luo SS, Ishibashi O, Ishikawa G, Ishikawa T, Katayama A, Mishima T, et al. Human villous trophoblasts express and secrete placenta-specific microRNAs into maternal circulation via exosomes. Biology of reproduction. 2009;81 (4):717-29. Epub 2009/06/06.

[26] Redman CW, Tannetta DS, Dragovic RA, Gardiner C, Southcombe JH, Collett GP, et al. Review: Does size matter? Placental debris and the pathophysiology of pre-eclampsia. Placenta. 2012;33 Suppl:S48-54. Epub 2012/01/06.

[27] Hegmans JP, Bard MP, Hemmes A, Luider TM, Kleijmeer MJ, Prins JB, et al. Proteomic analysis of exosomes secreted by human mesothelioma cells. The American journal of pathology. 2004;164 (5):1807-15. Epub 2004/04/28.

[28] Welton JL, Khanna S, Giles PJ, Brennan P, Brewis IA, Staffurth J, et al. Proteomics analysis of bladder cancer exosomes. Molecular & cellular proteomics : MCP. 2010;9 (6):1324-38. Epub 2010/03/13.

[29] Pisitkun T, Gandolfo MT, Das S, Knepper MA, Bagnasco SM. Application of systems biology principles to protein biomarker discovery: Urinary exosomal proteome in renal transplantation. Proteomics Clinical applications. 2012;6 (5- 6):268 78. Epub 2012/05/30.

[30] Gonzales PA, Pisitkun T, Hoffert JD, Tchapyjnikov D, Star RA, Kleta R, et al. Large-scale proteomics and phosphoproteomics of urinary exosomes. Journal of the American Society of Nephrology : JASN. 2009;20 (2):363-79. Epub 2008/12/06.

[31] Li Y, Zhang Y, Qiu F, Qiu Z. Proteomic identification of exosomal LRG1: a potential urinary biomarker for detecting NSCLC. Electrophoresis. 2011;32 (1 5):1976-83. Epub 2011/05/11.

[32] Zhang Y, Li Y, Qiu F, Qiu Z. Comprehensive analysis of low-abundance proteins in human urinary exosomes using peptide ligand library technology, peptide OFFGEL fractionation and nanoHPLC-chip-MS/MS. Electrophoresis. 2010;31 (23-2 4):3797-807. Epub 2010/11/18.

[33] Laulagnier K, Motta C, Hamdi S, Roy S, Fauvelle F, Pageaux JF, et al. Mast cell- and dendritic cell-derived exosomes display a specific lipid composition and an unusual

membrane organization. The Biochemical journal. 2004;380(Pt 1):161-71. Epub 2004/02/18.

[34] Wubbolts R, Leckie RS, Veenhuizen PT, Schwarzmann G, Mobius W, Hoernschemeyer J, et al. Proteomic and biochemical analyses of human B cell-derived exosomes. Potential implications for their function and multivesicular body formation. The Journal of biological chemistry. 2003;278 (1 3):10963-72. Epub 2003/01/10.

[35] Keller S, Sanderson MP, Stoeck A, Altevogt P. Exosomes: from biogenesis and secretion to biological function. Immunology letters. 2006;107 (2):102-8. Epub 2006/10/28.

[36] Raposo G, Nijman HW, Stoorvogel W, Liejendekker R, Harding CV, Melief CJ, et al. B lymphocytes secrete antigen-presenting vesicles. The Journal of experimental medicine. 1996;183 (3):1161-72. Epub 1996/03/01.

[37] Denzer K, van Eijk M, Kleijmeer MJ, Jakobson E, de Groot C, Geuze HJ. Follicular dendritic cells carry MHC class II-expressing microvesicles at their surface. J Immunol. 2000;165 (3):1259-65. Epub 2000/07/21.

[38] Clayton A, Court J, Navabi H, Adams M, Mason MD, Hobot JA, et al. Analysis of antigen presenting cell derived exosomes, based on immuno-magnetic isolation and flow cytometry. Journal of immunological methods. 2001;247 (1- 2):163-74. Epub 2001/01/11.

[39] Laulagnier K, Vincent-Schneider H, Hamdi S, Subra C, Lankar D, Record M. Characterization of exosome subpopulations from RBL-2H3 cells using fluorescent lipids. Blood cells, molecules & diseases. 2005;35 (2):116-21. Epub 2005/07/19.

[40] Denzer K, Kleijmeer MJ, Heijnen HF, Stoorvogel W, Geuze HJ. Exosome: from internal vesicle of the multivesicular body to intercellular signaling device. Journal of cell science. 2000;113 Pt 19:3365-74. Epub 2000/09/14.

[41] Mathivanan S, Fahner CJ, Reid GE, Simpson RJ. ExoCarta 2012: database of exosomal proteins, RNA and lipids. Nucleic acids research. 2012;40(Database issue):D1241-4. Epub 2011/10/13.

[42] Tauro BJ, Greening DW, Mathias RA, Ji H, Mathivanan S, Scott AM, et al. Comparison of ultracentrifugation, density gradient separation, and immunoaffinity capture methods for isolating human colon cancer cell line LIM1863-derived exosomes. Methods. 2012;56 (2):293-304. Epub 2012/01/31.

[43] Taylor DD, Zacharias W, Gercel-Taylor C. Exosome isolation for proteomic analyses and RNA profiling. Methods Mol Biol. 2011;728:235-46. Epub 2011/04/07.

[44] Taylor DD, Akyol S, Gercel-Taylor C. Pregnancy-associated exosomes and their modulation of T cell signaling. J Immunol. 2006;176 (3):1534-42. Epub 2006/01/21.

[45] Thery C, Amigorena S, Raposo G, Clayton A. Isolation and characterization of exosomes from cell culture supernatants and biological fluids. Current protocols in cell

biology / editorial board, Juan S Bonifacino (et al). 2006;Chapter 3:Unit 3 22. Epub 2008/01/30.

[46] Yamada T, Inoshima Y, Matsuda T, Ishiguro N. Comparison of Methods for Isolating Exosomes from Bovine Milk. The Journal of veterinary medical science / the Japanese Society of Veterinary Science. 2012. Epub 2012/07/13.

[47] Deatherage BL, Cookson BT. Membrane vesicle release in bacteria, eukaryotes, and archaea: a conserved yet underappreciated aspect of microbial life. Infection and immunity. 2012;80 (6):1948-57. Epub 2012/03/14.

[48] Southcombe J, Tannetta D, Redman C, Sargent I. The immunomodulatory role of syncytiotrophoblast microvesicles. PloS one. 2011;6 (5):e20245. Epub 2011/06/03.

[49] Bobrie A, Colombo M, Raposo G, Thery C. Exosome secretion: molecular mechanisms and roles in immune responses. Traffic. 2011;12 (1 2):1659-68. Epub 2011/06/08.

[50] Ambros V. The functions of animal microRNAs. Nature. 2004;431 (700 6):350-5. Epub 2004/09/17.

[51] Zhang HC, Liu XB, Huang S, Bi XY, Wang HX, Xie LX, et al. Microvesicles derived from human umbilical cord mesenchymal stem cells stimulated by hypoxia promote angiogenesis both in vitro and in vivo. Stem cells and development. 2012. Epub 2012/07/31.

[52] Zhang HG, Zhuang X, Sun D, Liu Y, Xiang X, Grizzle WE. Exosomes and immune surveillance of neoplastic lesions: a review. Biotechnic & histochemistry : official publication of the Biological Stain Commission. 2012;87 (3):161-8. Epub 2012/01/06.

[53] Mincheva-Nilsson L, Nagaeva O, Chen T, Stendahl U, Antsiferova J, Mogren I, et al. Placenta-derived soluble MHC class I chain-related molecules down-regulate NKG2D receptor on peripheral blood mononuclear cells during human pregnancy: a possible novel immune escape mechanism for fetal survival. J Immunol. 2006;176 (6):3585-92. Epub 2006/03/07.

[54] Lotvall J, Valadi H. Cell to cell signalling via exosomes through esRNA. Cell adhesion & migration. 2007;1 (3):156-8. Epub 2007/07/01.

[55] Vrijsen KR, Sluijter JP, Schuchardt MW, van Balkom BW, Noort WA, Chamuleau SA, et al. Cardiomyocyte progenitor cell-derived exosomes stimulate migration of endothelial cells. Journal of cellular and molecular medicine. 2010;14 (5):1064-70. Epub 2010/05/15.

[56] Breving K, Esquela-Kerscher A. The complexities of microRNA regulation: mirandering around the rules. The international journal of biochemistry & cell biology. 2010;42 (8):1316-29. Epub 2009/10/06.

[57] Rottiers V, Naar AM. MicroRNAs in metabolism and metabolic disorders. Nature reviews Molecular cell biology. 2012;13 (4):239-50. Epub 2012/03/23.

[58] Poy MN, Eliasson L, Krutzfeldt J, Kuwajima S, Ma X, Macdonald PE, et al. A pancreatic islet-specific microRNA regulates insulin secretion. Nature. 2004;432 (701 4): 226-30. Epub 2004/11/13.

[59] Guay C, Roggli E, Nesca V, Jacovetti C, Regazzi R. Diabetes mellitus, a microRNA-related disease? Translational research : the journal of laboratory and clinical medicine. 2011;157 (4):253-64. Epub 2011/03/23.

[60] Zampetaki A, Kiechl S, Drozdov I, Willeit P, Mayr U, Prokopi M, et al. Plasma microRNA profiling reveals loss of endothelial miR-126 and other microRNAs in type 2 diabetes. Circulation research. 2010;107 (6):810-7. Epub 2010/07/24.

[61] Costa SL, Proctor L, Dodd JM, Toal M, Okun N, Johnson JA, et al. Screening for placental insufficiency in high-risk pregnancies: is earlier better? Placenta. 2008;29 (1 2): 1034-40. Epub 2008/10/22.

[62] Cartwright JE, Fraser R, Leslie K, Wallace AE, James JL. Remodelling at the maternal-fetal interface: relevance to human pregnancy disorders. Reproduction. 2010;140 (6): 803-13. Epub 2010/09/15.

[63] Sobrevia L, Abarzua F, Nien JK, Salomon C, Westermeier F, Puebla C, et al. Review: Differential placental macrovascular and microvascular endothelial dysfunction in gestational diabetes. Placenta. 2011;32 Suppl 2:S159-64. Epub 2011/01/11.

[64] Cetkovic A, Miljic D, Ljubic A, Patterson M, Ghatei M, Stamenkovic J, et al. Plasma kisspeptin levels in pregnancies with diabetes and hypertensive disease as a potential marker of placental dysfunction and adverse perinatal outcome. Endocrine research. 2012;37 (2):78-88. Epub 2012/04/12.

[65] Taylor DD, Gercel-Taylor C. Exosomes/microvesicles: mediators of cancer-associated immunosuppressive microenvironments. Seminars in immunopathology. 2011;33 (5):441-54. Epub 2011/06/21.

[66] Chim SS, Shing TK, Hung EC, Leung TY, Lau TK, Chiu RW, et al. Detection and characterization of placental microRNAs in maternal plasma. Clinical chemistry. 2008;54 (3):482-90. Epub 2008/01/26.

[67] Miura K, Miura S, Yamasaki K, Higashijima A, Kinoshita A, Yoshiura K, et al. Identification of pregnancy-associated microRNAs in maternal plasma. Clinical chemistry. 2010;56 (1 1):1767-71. Epub 2010/08/24.

[68] Zhang Y, Fei M, Xue G, Zhou Q, Jia Y, Li L, et al. Elevated levels of hypoxia-inducible microRNA-210 in pre-eclampsia: new insights into molecular mechanisms for the disease. Journal of cellular and molecular medicine. 2012;16 (2):249-59. Epub 2011/03/11.

[69] Bullerdiek J, Flor I. Exosome-delivered microRNAs of "chromosome 19 microRNA cluster" as immunomodulators in pregnancy and tumorigenesis. Molecular cytogenetics. 2012;5 (1):27. Epub 2012/05/09.

[70] Zhao C, Dong J, Jiang T, Shi Z, Yu B, Zhu Y, et al. Early second-trimester serum miRNA profiling predicts gestational diabetes mellitus. PloS one. 2011;6 (8):e23925. Epub 2011/09/03.

[71] Donker RB, Mouillet JF, Chu T, Hubel CA, Stolz DB, Morelli AE, et al. The expression profile of C19MC microRNAs in primary human trophoblast cells and exosomes. Molecular human reproduction. 2012;18 (8):417-24. Epub 2012/03/03.

[72] Knight AM. Regulated release of B cell-derived exosomes: do differences in exosome release provide insight into different APC function for B cells and DC? European journal of immunology. 2008;38 (5):1186-9. Epub 2008/04/22.

[73] Soo CY, Song Y, Zheng Y, Campbell EC, Riches AC, Gunn-Moore F, et al. Nanoparticle tracking analysis monitors microvesicle and exosome secretion from immune cells. Immunology. 2012;136 (2):192-7. Epub 2012/02/22.

[74] Deng ZB, Poliakov A, Hardy RW, Clements R, Liu C, Liu Y, et al. Adipose tissue exosome-like vesicles mediate activation of macrophage-induced insulin resistance. Diabetes. 2009;58 (1 1):2498-505. Epub 2009/08/14.

[75] Sheng H, Hassanali S, Nugent C, Wen L, Hamilton-Williams E, Dias P, et al. Insulinoma-released exosomes or microparticles are immunostimulatory and can activate autoreactive T cells spontaneously developed in nonobese diabetic mice. J Immunol. 2011;187 (4):1591-600. Epub 2011/07/08.

[76] Boisvert MR, Koski KG, Skinner CD. Increased oxidative modifications of amniotic fluid albumin in pregnancies associated with gestational diabetes mellitus. Analytical chemistry. 2010;82 (3):1133-7. Epub 2010/01/13.

[77] Salem AH, Nosseir NS, El Badawi MG, Shoair MI, Fadel RA. Growth assessment of diabetic rat fetuses under the influence of insulin and melatonin: a morphologic study. Anthropologischer Anzeiger; Bericht uber die biologisch-anthropologische Literatur. 2010;68 (2):129-38. Epub 2010/01/01.

[78] Georgiou HM, Lappas M, Georgiou GM, Marita A, Bryant VJ, Hiscock R, et al. Screening for biomarkers predictive of gestational diabetes mellitus. Acta diabetologica. 2008;45 (3):157-65. Epub 2008/05/23.

[79] Metzger BE, Lowe LP, Dyer AR, Trimble ER, Chaovarindr U, Coustan DR, et al. Hyperglycemia and adverse pregnancy outcomes. The New England journal of medicine. 2008;358 (1 9):1991-2002. Epub 2008/05/09.

[80] Lindsay RS. Many HAPO returns: maternal glycemia and neonatal adiposity: new insights from the Hyperglycemia and Adverse Pregnancy Outcomes (HAPO) study. Diabetes. 2009;58 (2):302-3. Epub 2009/01/28.

[81] Biri A, Onan A, Devrim E, Babacan F, Kavutcu M, Durak I. Oxidant status in maternal and cord plasma and placental tissue in gestational diabetes. Placenta. 2006;27 (2-3):327-32. Epub 2005/12/13.

[82] Desoye G, Hauguel-de Mouzon S. The human placenta in gestational diabetes mellitus. The insulin and cytokine network. Diabetes care. 2007;30 Suppl 2:S120-6. Epub 2008/02/27.

[83] Taylor DD, Gercel-Taylor C. MicroRNA signatures of tumor-derived exosomes as diagnostic biomarkers of ovarian cancer. Gynecologic oncology. 2008;110 (1):13-21. Epub 2008/07/01.

[84] Hedlund M, Nagaeva O, Kargl D, Baranov V, Mincheva-Nilsson L. Thermal- and oxidative stress causes enhanced release of NKG2D ligand-bearing immunosuppressive exosomes in leukemia/lymphoma T and B cells. PloS one. 2011;6 (2):e16899. Epub 2011/03/03.

[85] Aoki N, Jin-no S, Nakagawa Y, Asai N, Arakawa E, Tamura N, et al. Identification and characterization of microvesicles secreted by 3T3-L1 adipocytes: redox- and hormone-dependent induction of milk fat globule-epidermal growth factor 8-associated microvesicles. Endocrinology. 2007;148 (8):3850-62. Epub 2007/05/05.

[86] Soderberg A, Barral AM, Soderstrom M, Sander B, Rosen A. Redox-signaling transmitted in trans to neighboring cells by melanoma-derived TNF-containing exosomes. Free radical biology & medicine. 2007;43 (1):90-9. Epub 2007/06/15.

[87] Eldh M, Ekstrom K, Valadi H, Sjostrand M, Olsson B, Jernas M, et al. Exosomes communicate protective messages during oxidative stress; possible role of exosomal shuttle RNA. PloS one. 2010;5 (1 2):e15353. Epub 2010/12/24.

[88] Barker DJ. In utero programming of cardiovascular disease. Theriogenology. 2000;53 (2):555-74. Epub 2000/03/29.

[89] Barker DJ. The origins of the developmental origins theory. Journal of internal medicine. 2007;261 (5):412-7. Epub 2007/04/21.

[90] Barker DJ, Gelow J, Thornburg K, Osmond C, Kajantie E, Eriksson JG. The early origins of chronic heart failure: impaired placental growth and initiation of insulin resistance in childhood. European journal of heart failure. 2010;12 (8):819-25. Epub 2010/05/28.

[91] Ehrlich SF, Crites YM, Hedderson MM, Darbinian JA, Ferrara A. The risk of large for gestational age across increasing categories of pregnancy glycemia. American journal of obstetrics and gynecology. 2011;204 (3):240 e1-6. Epub 2011/01/21.

[92] Rabinowits G, Gercel-Taylor C, Day JM, Taylor DD, Kloecker GH. Exosomal microRNA: a diagnostic marker for lung cancer. Clinical lung cancer. 2009;10 (1):42-6. Epub 2009/03/18.

[93] Roberson CD, Atay S, Gercel-Taylor C, Taylor DD. Tumor-derived exosomes as mediators of disease and potential diagnostic biomarkers. Cancer biomarkers : section A of Disease markers. 2010;8 (4- 5):281-91. Epub 2010/01/01.

[94] Gonzales PA, Zhou H, Pisitkun T, Wang NS, Star RA, Knepper MA, et al. Isolation and purification of exosomes in urine. Methods Mol Biol. 2010;641:89-99. Epub 2010/04/22.

[95] Chen X, Ba Y, Ma L, Cai X, Yin Y, Wang K, et al. Characterization of microRNAs in serum: a novel class of biomarkers for diagnosis of cancer and other diseases. Cell research. 2008;18 (1 0):997-1006. Epub 2008/09/04.

[96] Mitchell PS, Parkin RK, Kroh EM, Fritz BR, Wyman SK, Pogosova-Agadjanyan EL, et al. Circulating microRNAs as stable blood-based markers for cancer detection. Proceedings of the National Academy of Sciences of the United States of America. 2008;105 (3 0):10513-8. Epub 2008/07/30.

[97] Gilad S, Meiri E, Yogev Y, Benjamin S, Lebanony D, Yerushalmi N, et al. Serum microRNAs are promising novel biomarkers. PloS one. 2008;3 (9):e3148. Epub 2008/09/06.

[98] Nilsson J, Skog J, Nordstrand A, Baranov V, Mincheva-Nilsson L, Breakefield XO, et al. Prostate cancer-derived urine exosomes: a novel approach to biomarkers for prostate cancer. British journal of cancer. 2009;100 (1 0):1603-7. Epub 2009/04/30.

[99] Keller S, Rupp C, Stoeck A, Runz S, Fogel M, Lugert S, et al. CD24 is a marker of exosomes secreted into urine and amniotic fluid. Kidney international. 2007;72 (9): 1095-102. Epub 2007/08/19.

[100] Biancone L, Bruno S, Deregibus MC, Tetta C, Camussi G. Therapeutic potential of mesenchymal stem cell-derived microvesicles. Nephrology, dialysis, transplantation : official publication of the European Dialysis and Transplant Association - European Renal Association. 2012;27 (8):3037-42. Epub 2012/08/02.

[101] Gatti S, Bruno S, Deregibus MC, Sordi A, Cantaluppi V, Tetta C, et al. Microvesicles derived from human adult mesenchymal stem cells protect against ischaemia-reperfusion-induced acute and chronic kidney injury. Nephrology, dialysis, transplantation : official publication of the European Dialysis and Transplant Association - European Renal Association. 2011;26 (5):1474-83. Epub 2011/02/18.

Chapter 4

The Adenosine–Insulin Signaling Axis in the Fetoplacental Endothelial Dysfunction in Gestational Diabetes

Enrique Guzmán-Gutiérrez, Pablo Arroyo,
Fabián Pardo, Andrea Leiva and Luis Sobrevia

Additional information is available at the end of the chapter

http://dx.doi.org/10.5772/55627

1. Introduction

Gestational diabetes (GD) is a syndrome associated with maternal hyperglycaemia and defective insulin signaling in the placenta (Metzger et al., 2007; Colomiere et al., 2009; ADA 2012). GD have been associated with abnormal fetal development and perinatal complications such as macrosomia, neonatal hypoglicaemia, and neurological disorders (Nold & Georgieff, 2004; Pardo et al., 2012). The main risk factor to predict the GD development are increased maternal age, overweight before pregnancy, a history of GD in the first pregnancy and history of intolerance abnormal D-glucose (Morisset et al., 2010). Clinical manifestations of GD have been atribuited to conditions of hyperglicaemia, hyperlipidemia, hyperinsulinemia, and fetal endothelial dysfunction (Nold & Goergieff, 2004; Greene & Solomon, 2005; Sobrevia et al., 2011). Moreover, GD produces alterations in vascular reactivity (i.e., endothelium dependent vasodilation), which is considered a marker of endothelial dysfunction (De Vriese et al., 2000; Sobrevia et al., 2011; Westermeier et al., 2011; Salomón et al., 2012).

2. Gestational diabetes effect on endothelial function

GD generates structural and funtional alterations, including placental microvascular and macrovascular endothelial disfunction (Tchirikov et al., 2002; Biri et al., 2006; Sobrevia et al., 2011), observations showing an altered regulation of vascular tone in the fetal-placental circulation (San Martín & Sobrevia, 2006; Casanello et al., 2007; Sobrevia et al., 2011). The distal segment of umbilical cord and the placenta correspond to vascular beds without innervation (Marzioni et al., 2004), therefore local regulation of vascular tone results from a balanced combination of the synthesis, release and bioactivity endothelium-derived vasodilators (i.e., nitric oxide (NO), prostanglandins, adenosine) and vasoconstrictors (i.e., endothelin-1, angiotensin II) (Olsson & Pearson, 1990; Becker et al., 2000). It was reported that arteries and veins in the human placenta from pregnancies with GD have an increase in NO synthesis (Figueroa et al., 2000). Furthermore, the same result was obtained from primary cultures of human umbilical vein endothelial cells (HUVEC) from pregnant women diagnosed with GD (Sobrevia et al., 1995). Therefore, vascular disfunction resulting from GD may result from a functional dissociation between NO synthesis and its bioavailability in the human placental circulation (Sobrevia et al., 2011). Even when endothelial dysfunction is associated with GD, this is referred to as an alteration of NO synthesis and the uptake of cationic aminoacid L-arginine (i.e., L-arginine/NO pathway) (Figure 1) and a lack of mechanism behind these effects of GD is still a reality (Pardo et al., 2012). However, it is accepted that GD is a result of multiple mechanisms of metabolic alteration, including human fetal endothelial sensitivity to vasoactive molecules such as adenosine (Vásquez et al., 2004; San Martín & Sobrevia, 2006; Sobrevia et al., 2011; Pardo et al., 2012).

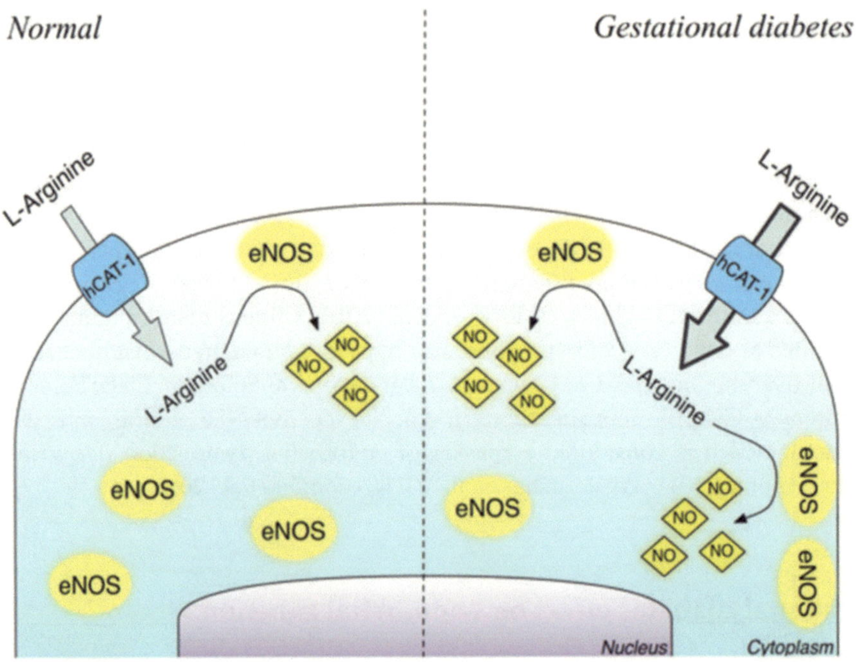

Figure 1. Fetal endothelial dysfunction in gestational diabetes. Human umbilical vein endothelial cells (HUVEC) from gestational diabetes (*Gestational diabetes*) exhibit increased human cationic amino acids transporter 1 (hCAT-1)–mediated L-arginine transport and endothelial nitric oxide synthase (eNOS)-dependent nitric oxide (NO) synthesis compared with HUVEC from normal pregnancies (*Normal*). From Vásquez et al (2004), San Martín & Sobrevia (2006), Westermeier et al (2011).

3. L–arginine transport in endotelial cells

L-arginine transport in human cells corresponding to different system of amino acids transports, someone of them, it is y^+ system (high affinity, sodium independent) and sodium dependent ($b^{0,+}$, $B^{0,+}$, e y^+L) (San Martín & Sobrevía, 2006; Wu, 2009). System y^+ has for five cationic amino acids transporters (CAT): CAT1, CAT2A, CAT2B, CAT3 and CAT4 (Closs et al., 2006; Grillo et al., 2008), considered the main L-arginine transport mechanism in different cell types (Tong & Barbul, 2004). In addition, CAT-1 isoform is the main L-arginine transporter in the placenta (Table 1) (Grillo et al., 2008).

4. Human cationic amino acids transporter 1

Human CAT-1 (hCAT-1) expression is modulated by citokines (i.e., TNFα, TGFβ) (Irie et al., 1997; Visigalli et al., 2007; Vásquez et al., 2007) and hormones (i.e., insulin) (Simmons et al., 1996; González et al., 2004, 2011a). The gene coding for this protein is called *SLC7A1* and it was originally located on chromosome 13q12-q14 (Albritton et al., 1992; Hammermann et al., 2001) and now referred as 13q12.3 (Gene ID: 6541). This gene is formed by 13 exons and 11 introns, where exons -1 and -2 are untranslatable (Hammermann et al., 2001; Sobrevia & González 2009) and located at the start transcription in +1 exon (Sobrevia & González 2009, González et al., 2011a). hCAT1 is pH and sodium independent (Devés & Boyd, 1998; Cloos et al., 2006) with values for apparent K_m are between 100 and 150 μM, and subjected to *trans*-stimulation (uptake increased by its substrates at the *trans* side of the plasma membrane) (Cloos et al., 2006).

5. hCAT–1 mediated L–arginine transport regulation

L-Arginine transport via hCAT-1 is regulated by different conditions (Sobrevia & González, 2009; González et al., 2011a). In HUVEC, hCAT-1 expression increases by tumoral necreosis factor alpha (TNF-α) (Irie et al., 1997; Visigalli et al., 2007) and transforming growth factor beta (TGF-β) (Vásquez et al., 2007), in the presence of free radicals such as superoxide anion (O_2^-) (González et al., 2011b), insulin (González et al., 2011a; Guzmán-Gutiérrez et al., 2012a), activation of A_{2A} adenosine receptors (A_{2A}AR) (Vásquez et al., 2004; Guzmán-Gutiérrez et al., 2012a), or high extracelular D-glucose concentration (25 mM) (Vásquez et al., 2007). Interestingly, insulin, A_{2A}AR and extracellular D-glucose have been directly associated with GD (San Martín & Sobrevia, 2006). Notably, HUVEC from GD pregnancy have increased hCAT-1 expression (Vásquez et al., 2004). Moreover, oxidized low-density lipoprotein (oxLDL) and protein kinase C (PKC) activity increase this transporter abundance in the membrane in HEK293 (Zhang et al., 2008; Vina-Vilaseca et al., 2011). Based in a series of recetn publications (reviewed in Leiva et al., 2011; Sobrevia et al., 2011; Pardo et al., 2012) it is proposed that hCAT-1 mediated L-arginine transport in HUVEC from GD could depend on the regulation of *SLC7A1* gene expression.

6. Regulation of *SLC7A1* gene expression

The amino acid cationic transporters family are coding by *SLC7A* (1-4) gene (Verrey et al., 2004), where *SLC7A1* is coding for hCAT-1 (Hammermann et al., 2001). Among the genes coding for CAT-1 in rat, mouse and human there are several common characteristics, i.e., the promoter region lack TATA box, have multiple binding sites for specific protein 1 (Sp1) and have an extensive 3'-untranslated region (3'UTR) which could play roles in the regulation of RNA stability or translation (Aulak et al., 1996, 1999; Fernández et al., 2003; Hatzoglou et al., 2004). *SLC7A1* gene has multiple sites for diferent types of transcription factors such as nuclear factor κB (NF-κB) and Sp1, which is regulated by insulin or inflammatory processes (Sobrevia & González 2009). In HUVEC from normal pregnancies it has been described that insulin increased the *SLC7A1* transcriptional activity (González et al., 2011a; Guzmán-Gutiérrez et al., 2012a), a mechanism that is Sp1 dependent (between-177 and -105 pb from ATG), However, at present there are not studies in HUVEC from GD (Figure 2).

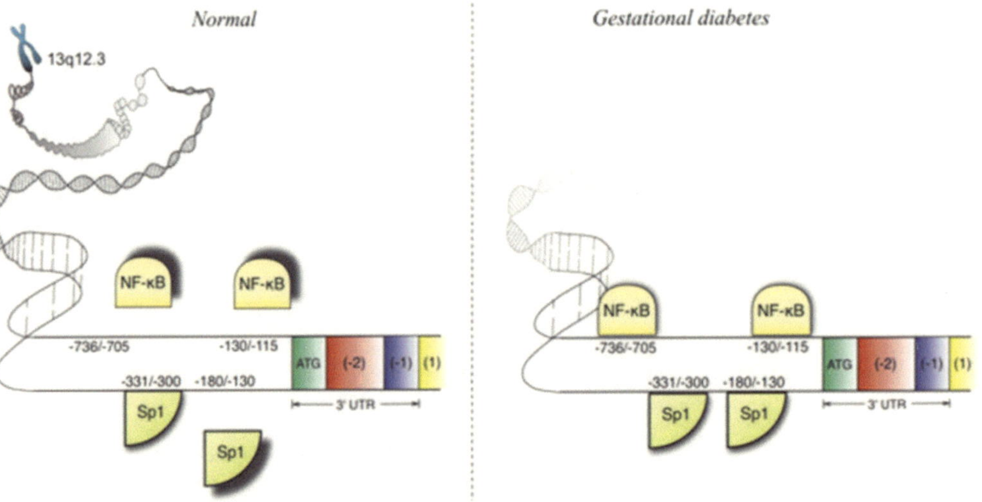

Figure 2. *SLC7A1* gene proximal promoter. The locus 13q12.3 codes for *SCL7A1*. In the proximal promoter of *SLC7A1* there are several consensus sequences for transcription factors, including the nuclear factor κB (NF-κB) and specific protein 1 (Sp1) between -115 and -736 pb from the transcriptional start point (ATG). In HUVEC from gestational diabetes (*Gestational diabetes*) NF-κB and Sp1 could bind to *SLC7A1* proximal promoter inducing its transcriptional activity. However, in HUVEC from normal pregnancies (*Normal*) basal transcriptional activity is commanded mainly by Sp1. The *SLC7A1* contains an ATG within the untranslatable region (3'-UTR) and 2 exons (exon -2 and exon -1). This region could be involved in post-transcriptional regulation of hCAT-1 protein. (1) regards exon 1 of the translatable region. From Hammerman et al. (2001), Hatzoglou et al. (2004), Sobrevia & González (2009).

Specific protein 1 (Sp1). The transcriptional factor Sp1 belongs to the super family Sp/Krupel-like factor, which is divided into Sp subfamilies, with 8 members (Sp1-Sp8) and KLF subfamily, with 15 members (Solomon et al., 2008). Then, Sp subfamily is divided into 2 groups Sp1-Sp4 (604-785 amino acids) and Sp5-Sp8 (394-785 amino acids) (Solomon et al., 2008; Wierstra, 2008). Sp1 has several consensus sites for various kinases, including calmodulin kinase

(CaMK), casein kinases (CK), protein kinase A (PKA), PKC, and p44/42^{mapk} (Samsons et al., 2002; Sobrevia & González 2009). Interestingly, insulin increases Sp1 activity in HepG2 cells, where raised genes transcription such as plasminogen activator inhibitor 1 (Banfi et al., 2001) and Apo A1 lipoprotein (Murao et al., 1998, Lam et al., 2003). In addition, in the skeletal muscle L6 cell line it has been demonstrated that insulin increases PKC expression via a Sp1-independent mechanism (Horovitz-Fried et al., 2007).

Nuclear factor κB. Nuclear factor κB (NF-κB) participates in inflammation being a main element in many diseases whose activation is induced and is protein synthesis independent, requiring post-translational changes to migrate to the nucleus (Grimm et al., 1993). NF-κB was described as a transcriptional factor activated by several immunological stimules, for example, TNFα and LPS (Crisóstomo et al., 2008; Nakao et al., 2002), or interleukine 1 (IL-1) (Jung et al., 2002). NF-κB activity is related with inhibitor κB (IκB), which is an inhibitor when is attached to NF-κB (Baldwin, 1996). Hyperglicaemia increases NF-κB protein abundance in the nucleus in HUVEC, a PI3K/Akt mechanism dependent (Sheu et al., 2005). Insulin acting in a short time (30 minutes) inhibits NF-κB activations (Zhang et al., 2010). High D-glucose is associated with NF-κB activation in human aortic endothelial cells (HAEC), and bovine aortic endothelial cells (BAEC) (Mohan et al., 2003; Sobrevia & González 2009; González et al., 2011b). In BAEC, insulin blocks high D-glucose effects on NF-κB activity (Aljada et al., 2001). This insulin effect has been seen in mononuclear cells from obese subjects, who have an increase in NF-κB activity (Dandona et al., 2001). NF-κB is also regulated by A_{2A}AR activation leading to inhibition in HUVEC (Sands et al., 2004). In other hands, in astrocytes A_{2A}AR activation leads to increased NF-κB activity (Ke et al., 2009). Probably, NF-κB has different functions depending on the cell type. Futhermore, A_3AR activates NF-κB in thyroid carcinoma (Morello et al., 2009; Bar-Yehuda et al., 2008) and in mononuclear cells from rheumatoid arthritis patients (Fishman et al., 2006; Madi et al., 2007). NF-κB activity has been associated with cationic amino acid transporter 2B (CAT-2B) in human saphenous vascular endothelial cells (HSVEC) in response to TNFα (Visigalli et al., 2007). In animal models it has been demonstrated that mCAT-2B requires activation of NF-κB in macrophages (Huang et al., 2004), and that LPS increases mCAT2 levels via NF-κB in these cells (Tsai et al., 2006). In animal models of GD it has has been demonstrated that NF-κB inhibition leads to an increase in insulin sensitivity in cheeps skeletal muscle (Yan et al., 2010), and increases GLUT-4 expression in GD rat uterus. However, there is no information regarding the role of NF-κB in human tissues or cells from GD.

7. Gestational diabetes effect on L–arginine transport in HUVEC

It has been reported that NO levels in amniotic fluid (von Mandach et al., 2003) and NO synthesis in placental vein and artery (Figueroa et al., 2000) are increased in GD. Early studies in HUVEC from GD pregnancies show increased NO synthesis and L-arginine transport (Sobrevia et al., 1995, 1997). These results were associated with an increase in eNOS number of copies for mRNA, protein level and activity (Vásquez et al., 2004; Farías et al., 2006, 2010; Westermeier et al., 2011). Moreover, HUVEC from GD pregnancies exhibit a higher number of copies of mRNA for hCAT-1 (Vásquez et al., 2004). Interestingly, HUVEC incubated with high D-glucose show increased NO synthesis and intracellular cGMP levels (Sobrevia et al., 1997; González et al., 2004, 2011a). In this phenomenon a role has been proposed for cell signaling pathways including PKC and p44/p42^{mapk} (Montecinos et al., 2000; Flores et al., 2003). Thus, in GD there is an increase in NO level associated with an increase in hCAT-1 mediated L-arginine transport.

In HUVEC from GD pregnancies insulin reduces L-arginine transport-increased observed in this cells compared with HUVEC from normal pregnancies (Sobrevia et al., 1998). Moreover, it was observed that insulin reduce NO synthesis-increased (Sobrevia et al., 1998). Another vasoactive molecule, including adenosine, increases L-arginine transport and eNOS activity (Vásquez et al., 2004; San Martín & Sobrevia 2006; Farías et al., 2006, 2010; Westermeier et al., 2011). It was observated by assays *in vitro* that the adenosine level in the culture medium of HUVEC from GD pregnancies (2.5 μM) is higher that HUVEC from normal pregnancies (50 nM) (Vásquez et al., 2004; Westermeier et al., 2011). Moreover, in HUVEC from normal pregnancies incubated with nitrobenzylthioinosine (NBTI, equilibrative adenosine transporters inhibitor) exhibit increased L-arginine transport, a phenomenon blocked by antagonists of A_{2A}AR, indicating that elevated extracellular adenosine level and A_{2A}AR activation are factors involved in the stimulation of L-arginine transport by NBTI (San Martín & Sobrevia, 2006; Westermeier et al., 2009; Sobrevia et al., 2011).

8. Adenosine receptors

Adenosine is a purine nucleoside associated with several biological functions, such as nucleotides synthesis or cellular energetic metabolism (Eltzschig, 2009). Moreover, this nucleoside is a vasodilator in coronary, cerebral, and muscular circulation, in several conditions including hypoxia and exercise (Berne et al., 1983). Extracellular adenosine is a signaling molecule that activates adenosine receptors (ARs). ARs belonging purinergic receptor P1 family, are coupled to G-protein and only four subtypes ARs, A_1, A_{2A}, A_{2B} y A_3 have been described (Fredholm et al., 2001, 2007, 2011; Burnstock et al., 2006, 2010). ARs stimulation generates several biological effects which are related with the expression pattern and membrane disponibility in a certain cellular type or tissue (Liu et al., 2002; Wyatt et al., 2002; Feoktistov et al., 2002). The protein assembly exhibits a short N-terminal (7-13 amino acids) compared with the C-terminal (32-120 amino acids) (Burnstock, 2006). Humans ARs transmembrane domains have between 39–61% of identical sequence and 11-18% with P2 family (nucleotide receptors) (Burnstock, 2006). The A_1AR, A_{2A}AR y A_3AR are activated by adenosine at nanomolar concentration, while A_{2B}AR requires micromolar concentration for its activation (Fredholm et al., 2001; 2011; Schulte & Fredholm, 2003; Eltzschig, 2009; Mundell & Kelly, 2010). A_1AR and A_3AR are clasically associated with inhibitory signaling receptors coupled to G_i/G_o protein; however, A_{2A}AR and A_{2B}AR are associated with stimulatory signaling receptors coupled to G_s protein (Klinger et al., 2002).

ARs activation depends on the adenosine extracellular level, a characteristic that is mainly regulated by adenosine membrane transporters (Baldwin et al., 2004; Burnstock, 2006;

Westermeier et al., 2009; Burnstock et al., 2010; Sobrevia et al., 2011). In HUVEC and in human placental microvascular endothelial cells (hPMEC) the extracellular adenosine is taken up mainly via the equilibrative nucleoside transporters (ENTs) (Westermeier et al., 2009; 2011; Sobrevia et al., 2011; Salomón et al., 2012). Interestingly, the sodium dependent, concentrative nucleoside transporters (CNT) have not been described in HUVEC or hPMEC (Sobrevia et al., 2011; Pardo et al., 2012). Several studies have described endothelial effects of adenosine, including a rise in the oxygen demand/delivery relation in human heart due to $A_{2A}AR$ activation-associated vasodilation (Shryock et al., 1998; Sundell et al., 2003), or reduction on norepinephrine release and peripheral vascular resistance by A_1AR activation in rat sympathetic nerve (Burgdorf et al., 2001, 2005). A summary of the potential biological effects resulting from activation of ARs is given in Table 2.

9. Role of adenosine receptors in gestational diabetes

The vasodilatory effect of adenosine, which is endothelial-derived NO-dependent, is mediated by activation of ARs (Sobrevia & Mann, 1997; Edmunds & Marshall, 2003; Vásquez et al., 2004; San Martín & Sobrevia, 2006; Ray & Marshall, 2006; Casanello et al., 2007; Escudero et al., 2008, 2009; Westermeier et al., 2009; Sobrevia et al., 2011). This is also seen in primary cultures of HUVEC from GD (Vásquez et al., 2004; San Martín & Sobrevia, 2006; Casanello et al., 2007; Westermeier et al., 2009; Farías et al., 2006, 2010) or in HUVEC from normal pregnancies exposed to high D-glucose (Muñoz et al., 2006; Puebla et al., 2008). The functional link between adenosine and L-arginine/NO pathway in HUVEC has been referred as the ALANO signalling pathway (i.e., *Adenosine/L-Arginine/Nitric Oxide*) (San Martín & Sobrevia, 2006). This mechanism has been proposed as a key new element for a better understanding of the endothelial dysfunction in conditions of hyperglicaemia, such as that seen in GD (Figure 3) (Pandolfi & Di Pietro, 2010).

The increased activity of ALANO pathway in GD involves extracellular adenosine accumulation resulting from reduced of adenosine uptake into endothelial cells (Vásquez et al., 2004; Farías et al., 2006, 2010). This means that changes in plasma adenosine concentration in the fetoplacental circulation could result in an altered blood flux control in the human placenta (Westermeier et al., 2009; Sobrevia et al., 2011). It was demonstrated that resistance of umbilical vessels from GD do not change with respect to vessels from normal pregnancies (Brown et al., 1990; Biri et al., 2006; Pietryga et al., 2006). It has been reported that plasma adenosine level in umbilical vein whole blood is higher in GD with respect to normal pregnancies (Westermeier et al., 2011). In addition, umbilical vein blood contained more adenosine compared with umbilical cord arteries in GD, thus suggestsing that an altered placental metabolism of this nucleoside is likely in this syndrome (Salomón et al., 2012). These results complement other studies showing increased adenosine concentration in umbilical vein blood from GD compare to normal pregnancies (Maguire et al., 1998) or in the extracellular medium in primary cultures for HUVEC and hPMEC from GD (Vásquez et al., 2004; Farías et al., 2006, 2010; Westermeier et al., 2011; Salomón et al., 2012). Even when all these observation have been made, there is not a full consense between the findings showing increased plasma level of adenosine and

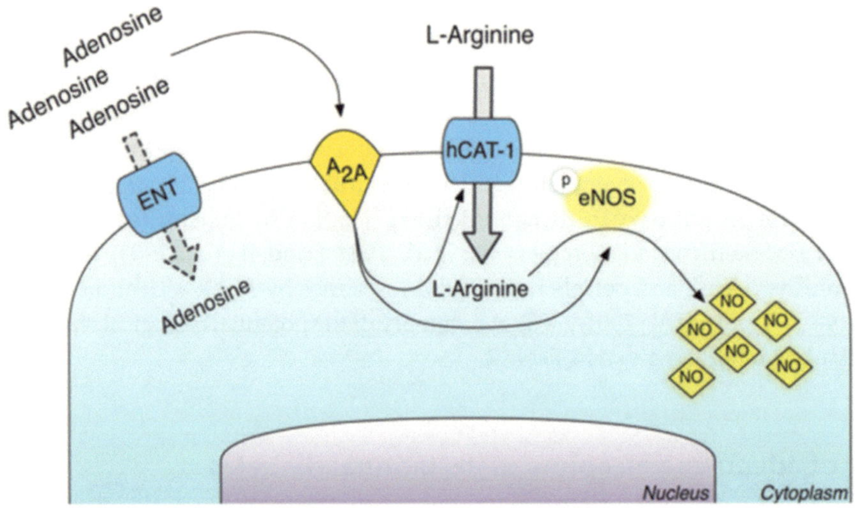

Figure 3. Endothelial ALANO pathway. The ALANO (*A*denosine/*L*-*A*rginine/*N*itric *o*xide) pathway is initiated by a low adenosine uptake via equilibrative nucleoside transporters (ENT) (dotted arrow) leading to increased extracellular adenosine concentration. Accumulation of adenosine activates A_{2A} adenosine receptors (A_{2A}) resulting in increased human cationic amino acid (hCAT-1)-mediated L-arginine transport and endothelial nitric oxide synthase (eNOS)-dependent nitric oxide (NO) synthesis. eNOS is activated by preferential Serine[1177] phosphorylation (p-eNOS). ALANO pathway has been associated as a new mechanism for the understanding of gestational diabetes effects on human fetal endothelial cells. From Vásquez et al. (2004), San Martín & Sobrevia (2006), Pandolfi & Di Pietro (2010).

endothelial dysfunction in GD pregnancies (Baldwin et al., 2004; San Martín & Sobrevia, 2006; Casanello et al., 2007; Westermeier et al., 2009; Sobrevia et al., 2011; Pardo et al., 2012).

10. Insulin

Insulin is a polypeptide hormone of 51 amino acid residues, synthesized and secreted by β cells in the Langerhans islets of pancreas as an inactive single polypeptide, i.e., preproinsulin, with an N-terminal signal sequence that determines its incorporation to secretory vesicles (Mounier et al., 2006). The proteolytic elimination of the signal sequence and the formation of three di-sulfur bridges yield the proinsulin. This molecule goes to the Golgi apparatus where it is modified and stored in secretory vesicles (Shepherd, 2004). The raise of D-glucose in the blood triggers insulin production through conversion of proinsulin to active insulin by proteases that will cut two peptide bonds to form the mature form of insulin in equimolar quantities of C peptide (Shepherd, 2004). Insulin is the archetypal growth hormone during fetal development, promotes the deposit of carbohydrates, lipids and protein in the tissues and D-glucose uptake. This hexose is the main source of energy in the fetus and its metabolism responds to fetal insulin since the 12th week of gestation (first trimester) (Desoye at al., 2007). Intracellular hormones and signals regulate insulin secretion, also the autonomous nervous system and the interaction of substrates like amino acids and mainly D-glucose (Shepherd,

2004). Once secreted from the pancreas, insulin exerts several effects on its target cells and regulates a myriad of processes in the organism (Muniyappa et al., 2007).

11. Role of insulin in gestational diabetes

The studies 'Summary and Recommendations of the Fourth International Workshop-Conference on Gestational Diabetes Mellitus' (Metzger & Coustan, 1998) and 'Gestational Diabetes Mellitus, Position Statement of the American Diabetes Association' (2004) list different priority areas regarding gestational diabetes research, proposing the characterization of regulatory mechanisms of fetal blood flow as a necessary attention sector, based in the lack of information about the effect of gestational diabetes over the fetoplacentary circulation. Furthermore, some reports (i.e., 'Summary and Recommendations of the Fifth International Workshop-Conference on Gestational Diabetes Mellitus') (Metzger et al., 2007) include recommendations for research in several aspects of placental function in the context of gestational diabetes. These recommendations include characterization of insulin resistant mechanisms and identification of cellular mechanism that reduces insulin signal in GD (Metzger et al., 2007). Although the role of insulin is accepted in GD, cellular signaling and the fetoplacental tissue response to insulin in this syndrome is not well understood (Hiden et al., 2009; Westermeier et al., 2009; Sobrevia & González, 2009; Sobrevia et al., 2009). Even when insulin receptors are expressed in human placental vasculature (Hiden et al., 2009; Westermeier et al., 2011; Salomón et al., 2012), there is limited information available about the biological action of insulin receptors activation and the vascular effects of insulin in the placental circulation in GD (Desoye & Hauguel-de Mouson, 2007; Barret et al., 2009; Genua et al., 2009; Sobrevia et al., 2011).

GD leads to abnormalities in the transplacental transport, an event that happens, among others factors, due to a lost in the hormonal balance induced by changes in the synthesis and signaling of insulin (Kuzuya & Matsuda, 1997; Metzger & Custan, 1998; Greene & Solomon, 2005; Biri et al., 2006; Sobrevia & González, 2009; Barret et al., 2009). Insulin causes vasodilation in normal subjects via a mechanism that is dependent on endothelium-derived NO (Steinberg & Baron, 2002; Sundell & Knuuti, 2003; Barret et al., 2009; Sonne et al., 2010; Timmerman et al., 2010). Furthermore, *in vitro* studies show that insulin activates L-arginine/NO signaling pathway in HUVEC (González et al., 2004, 2011a; Muñoz et al. 2006), hPMEC (Salomón et al., 2012) and in other endothelia (Sundell & Knuuti, 2003; Barrett et al., 2009). Initial observations suggested a differential vasodilatory effect of insulin between the macro and microvasculature of the human placenta from fetuses that were appropriate (AGA) or large (LGA) for gestational age in GD (Jo et al., 2009). This study shows that insulin-associated vasodilation depends on endothelium-derived NO in umbilical arteries and veins from normal pregnancies or GD, and that insulin did not alter chorionic vessels of normal pregnancies, but generated chorionic vessel relaxation in pregnancies with this syndrome. These observations were accompanied by increased level of insulin in the plasma from umbilical cord blood, confirming earlier observations (Westgate et al., 2006; Lindsay et al., 2007; Colomiere et al., 2009). Interestingly, there is not information regarding the potential mechanism(s) associated with this specific response to insulin by the fetoplacental unit in GD (Youngren et al., 2007, Barrett et al., 2009; Sobrevia & González, 2009; Sobrevia et al., 2011).

12. hCAT–1–mediated L–arginine transport regulated by insulin

In primary cultures of HUVEC in euglycemia conditions (i.e., containing 5 mM D-glucose) and in the presence of physiological concentrations of insulin (0.1-1 nM) it has been observed an increase of the maximum velocity of L-arginine transport (V_{max}), with no significant changes in the apparent K_m (González et al., 2004). This phenomenon was seen in a higher maximum transport capacity (i.e., V_{max}/K_m) (Casanello et al., 2007; Vásquez et al., 2004; Escudero et al., 2008). The reported magnitude of stimulatory effect of L-arginine transport (~5 fold) was comparable to *trans*-stimulation with lysine of L-arginine uptake (González et al., 2004). These results are complemented by an increased number of copies of mRNA for hCAT1 (González et al., 2004) and protein abundance (González et al., 2011a; Guzmán-Gutiérrez et al., 2012a). These studies suggest that L-arginine transport is stimulated by insulin by increasing the expression of hCAT1 in HUVEC (Sobrevia & González, 2009). Furthermore, it has been proposed that the effect of insulin on transport of L-arginine is a cellular signaling mechanism including phosphatidylinositol 3 kinase (PI3K), protein kinase C (PKC) and mitogen-activated protein kinases p44 and p42 ($p42/p44^{mapk}$) (González et al., 2004). This phenomenon will increase the binding of Sp1 to *SLC7A1* promoter in the consensus area between -177 to -105 bp from the ATG (González et al., 2011) (Figure 4). Furthermore, in HUVEC from pregnancies with GD in the presence of 5 mM D-glucose, insulin (1 nM) decreases overall L-arginine transport, whereas in 25 mM D-glucose, insulin insensitivity is seen (0.1-10 nM) (Sobrevia et al., 1996, 1998). These findings open the option of studying a mechanism of insulin resistance mediated by insulin receptor or post-insulin receptor defects. Recently it has been reported that HUVEC (Westermeier et al., 2011) and hPMEC (Salomón et al., 2012) express at least two insulin receptor subtypes, IR type A (IR-A) and IR type B (IR-B). In HUVEC from GD the IR-A/IR-B ratio is 1.6 fold compared with cells from normal pregnanices, an effect due to increased IR-A mRNA expression. However, in hPMEC from GD pregnancies the IR-A mRNA expression was reduced, while IR-B mRNA expression was increased compared with cells from normal pregnancies. Thus, a differential and cell specific involvement of these IR subtypes in GD and perhaps other pathologies of pregnancy, such as pre-eclampsia (Mate et al., 2012) could occur.

13. Insulin receptors

Insulin generates its biological effects via activation of insulin receptors in the plasma membrane of endothelial cells of human umbilical vein (Zheng & Quon, 1996; Nitert et al., 2005) and placental microvasculature (Desoye & Hauguel-de Mouzon, 2007; Hiden et al., 2009). The gene coding the human insulin receptor is located on the short arm of chromosome 19 and consists of 22 exons and 21 introns (Seino et al., 1989). The mature insulin receptor is a glycoprotein composed of two β subunits (transmembrane domain) joined by disulfide

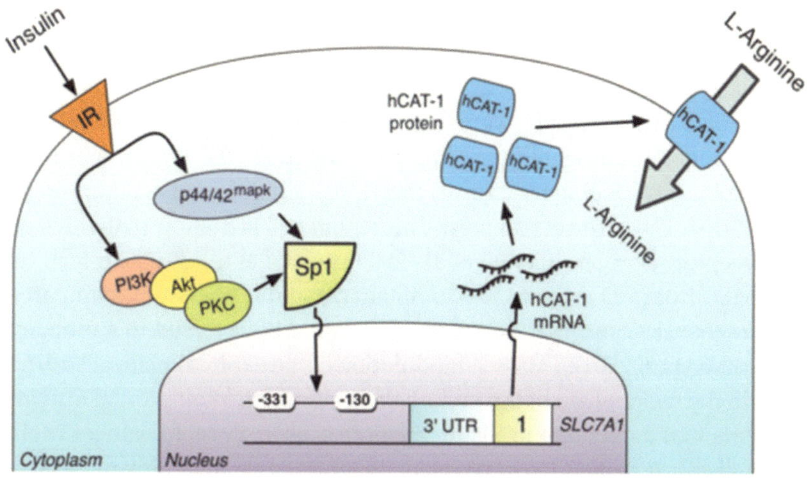

Figure 4. Insulin modulation of hCAT-1 mediated L-arginine transport in HUVEC. Insulin activates insulin receptors (IR) trigerring signaling cascades involving phosphoinositol 3 kinase (PI3K), Akt and protein kinases C (PKC), and in parallel p44 and p42 mitogen-activated protein kinases ($p44/42^{mapk}$). These molecules induce an increase in Sp1 cytoplasm levels, which then promotes *SLC7A1* transcriptional activity due to higher Sp1 activity (between the region -331 to -130 bp from the transctiptional start point (3'UTR)) leading to an increase in the hCAT-1 mRNA expression and protein abundance at the plasma membrane allowing higher L-arginine uptake. From González et al. (2004, 2011).

bridges. The *N*-terminal extracellular α-subunit (exons 1-2) and the cysteine-rich domain (exons 3-5) are responsible for the high affinity for the insulin in combination with *C*-terminal domain (amino acid residues 704-719) (Kristensen et al., 1998; Thørsoe et al., 2010). Insulin signaling involves the participation of PI3K as regulatory protein of D-glucose metabolism in tissues such as skeletal muscle and adipocytes promoting translocation of isoform 4 of D-glucose transporter (GLUT4) to the plasma membrane and stimulating NO production and endothelium-dependent vasodilation (Bergandi et al., 2003). The mitogenic effect is primarily mediated by MAPK, which regulates the growth, differentiation and control, for example, the synthesis of vasoconstrictor molecules such as ET-1 (Kim et al., 2006; Muniyappa et al., 2007).

With the cloning of the two isoforms of the insulin receptor, i.e., IR-A and IR-B, it the possibility of a differential response to insulin by selective activation (or semi selective) of these isoforms has been proposed (Ullrich et al., 1985; Ebina et al., 1985; Frasca et al., 1999; Sesti et al., 2001; Belfiore et al., 2009; Genua et al., 2009; Sciacca et al., 2003, 2010; Thørsoe et al., 2010; Sen et al., 2010; Westermeier et al., 2011; Sobrevia et al., 2011; Leiva et al., 2011; Pardo et al., 2012; Salomón et al., 2012). The IR-A cDNA (exon 11-) lacks exon 11, and IR-B (exon 11+) contains exon 11 (Genua et al., 2009; Thørsoe et al., 2010; Sen et al., 2010). Both isoforms are expressed in insulin-sensitive tissues (liver, muscle and adipose tissue) (Moller et al., 1989; Mosthaf et al., 1990), but IR-A is predominantly expressed in the fetus and placenta, where it plays a role in embryonic development (Frasca et al., 1999). These isoforms are also expressed in adult tissue, especially in the brain (Belfiore et al., 2009). Moreover, IR-B is expressed mainly in differentiated adult tissues, such as the liver, and associates with increased metabolic effects of insulin (Sciacca et al., 2003, 2010; Genua et al., 2009; Sen et al., 2010). Dysregulation of the insulin receptor splicing in key tissues responsive to insulin may occur in patients with insulin resistance, but this role is unclear in diabetes mellitus (Belfiore et al., 2009) and not reported in GD (Sobrevia et al., 2011; Leiva et al., 2011; Pardo et al., 2012). A recent study shows that IR-A activation by insulin activates a predominant metabolic signaling pathway (p42/p44^{mapk}/Akt activity ratio >1) instead of a predominant mitogenic signaling pathway (p42/p44^{mapk}/Akt activity ratio <1), as described in response to IR-B activation in the R- cell line of mouse embryonic fibroblasts (Sciacca et al., 2010). These results suggest differential cell signaling pathways activated by these insulin receptor subtypes (Genua et al., 2009; Sciacca et al., 2010). In fact, recently was shown that hPMEC from GD exhibit a predominant metabolic phenotype compared with cells from normal pregnancies, and that this phenotype could be reversed to a mitogenic, normal phenotype (Salomón et al., 2012). Thus, a modulation of the expression level will, perhaps, has a consequence in the metabolism of the endothelial cells of the fetoplacental unit in GD. Other evidence suggests that a decrease in insulin response, as in Type 2 Diabetes Mellitus where the predominant isoform is IR-A (Norgren et al., 1994), and in states of insulin resistance where IR-A/IR-B increases in the skeletal muscle of patients with myotonic dystrophy type 1 (Savkur et al., 2001) and 2 (Savkur et al., 2001; Phillips et al., 1998).

Insulin, insulin-like growth factor 1 (IGF1) and 2 (IGF2) generate various metabolic and mitogenic effects through activation of receptors associated with tyrosine kinase activity on the surface of the target cells. These hormones have high structural homology. The two receptors may act as ligands for these molecules. At physiological concentrations insulin and IGF1 are attached only to the insulin and IGF receptors, respectively. While, IGF2 receptor binds to IGF1 (IGFR1) and IR-A (Frasca et al., 1999). The affinity of IGF2 by IR-A is less than that of insulin for this receptor (EC_{50} 0.9 versus 2.5 nM, respectively), while the binding of IGF1 to IR-A is very high (EC_{50}>30 nM). The affinity of IGF2 to IGFR1 is comparable to that of IGF1 (EC_{50} 0.6 versus 0.2 nM, respectively), where insulin binds weakly to this receptor (EC_{50}>30 nM) (Pandini et al., 2002). Therefore, there may be a differential response to insulin in the fetoplacental vasculature given by preferential activation of one insulin receptor subtype in pregnancies with GD.

14. Insulin effects are modulated by adenosine

Insulin sensitivity is increased in rats supplemented with adenosine in the diet (Ardiansyah et al., 2010). These data are complemented by similar observations described in diabetic rat adipocytes (Joost & Steinfelder, 1982), nondiabetic rat skeletal muscle (Vergauwen et al., 1995), and patients with TIDM who received an infusion of adenosine (Srinivasan et al., 2005) (Table 3). In other studies, adenosine, agonists and antagonists concentration of adenosine receptors, and insulin used was greater than 100 nM, suggesting for adenosine receptors, that the activation and inhibition of this receptors was complete, and for insulin, involving IR-A, IR-B, and IGF receptors in the system. However, in some studies the concentration of insulin that was used is relatively selective for the receptors of insulin, suggesting the possibility that activation of adenosine receptors increases insulin effect (Webster et al., 1996; Ciaraldi et al., 1997; Sundell et al., 2002; Srinivasan et al., 2005). Similarly, oyther groups show that inhibition of adenosine receptors blocks the effect of insulin mediated only by the insulin receptor (Pawelczyk et al.,

http://dx.doi.org/10.5772/55627

2005; Dhalla et al., 2008). Moreover, the expression and activation of adenosine receptors reduces plasma levels of D-glucose, due to increased release and the biological effect of insulin in diabetic rats (Johansson et al., 2006; Németh et al., 2007; Töpfer et al., 2008). Activation of A_1AR (Vergauwen et al., 1994) or decreased expression A_{2B}AR (Ardiansyah et al., 2010; Figler et al., 2011), results in an increased sensitivity to insulin, but there is no information about the specific mechanisms explaining the biological actions of adenosine (Burnstock et al., 2006; San Martín & Sobrevia, 2006; Mundell & Kelly, 2010). The activation of the A_{2B}AR, but to a lesser degree than the A_1AR, prevents the development of diabetes in mouse (Németh et al., 2007). However, a study in C57BL/6J mice suggests that insulin sensitivity decreases by activation of A_{2B}AR, except in the knockout mouse for this receptor, suggesting that A_{2B}AR is involved in the phenomenon of insulin resistance (Figler et al., 2011). This finding opens the possibility that the increase and/or inhibition of the expression or activity of ARs may be associated as a protective mechanism against this syndrome. Recently, we have published that A_{2A}AR activation in HUVEC from normal pregnancies modulate insulin effect on hCAT-1-mediated L-arginine transport and expression (Guzmán-Gutiérrez et al., 2012a). Interestingly, we saw that in HUVEC from GD insulin reversed GD-increased hCAT-1-mediated L-arginine transport, a mechanism that is dependent on A_1AR activation (Guzmán-Gutiérrez et al., 2012b). Based on these findings, a possible cross talk between the adenosine receptors and insulin receptors is feasible. This phenomenon could create a potential regulatory mechanism of the biological actions of insulin in the fetoplacental vasculature in GD (Figure 5).

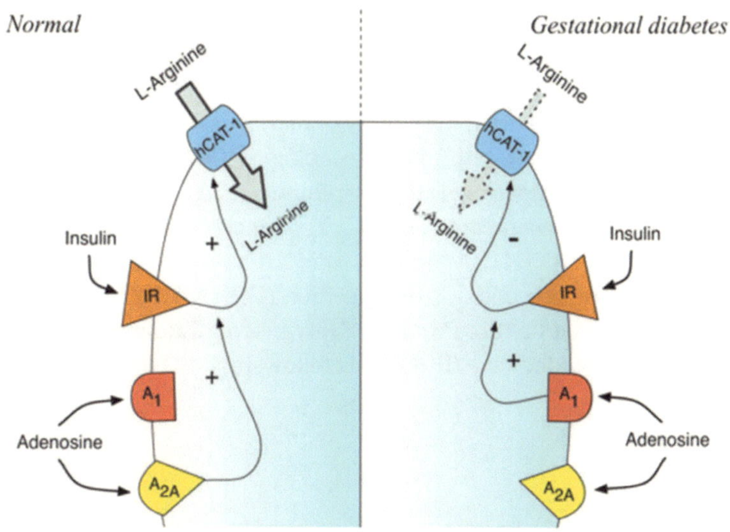

Figure 5. Adenosine/insulin signaling axis involvement in the L-arginine transport in HUVEC. Insulin acting via insulin receptors (IR) increases (+) human cationic amino acid (hCAT-1)-mediated L-arginine transport in HUVEC from normal pregnancies (*Normal*). This biological action of insulin requires (+) activation of A_{2A} (A_{2A}), but not on A_1 adenosine receptors (A_1) by adenosine. In HUVEC from gestational diabetes insulin decreases (–) the hCAT-1 mediated L-arginine transport (dotted arrow), which was elevated in cells from this syndrome to values in cells from normal pregnancies. This biological action of insulin requires (+) activation of A_1, but not on A_{2A} adenosine receptors by adenosine. From Guzmán-Gutiérrez et al. (2011, 2012a,b)

15. Concluding remarks

GD associates with endotelial dysfunction in the fetoplacental macro and microcirculation associated with an increase in NO synthesis and hCAT-1 mediated L-arginine transport. Hyperinsulinemia and high plasma adenosine in umbilical blood in GD, suggest the involvement of these molecules in this syndrome. $A_{2A}AR$ and insulin receptors increase hCAT-1 and eNOS activity and expression in HUVEC from normal, while HUVEC from GD, activation of $A_{2A}AR$ would be part of mechanism that explain the increase of NO synthesis (i.e., ALANO pathway). In other hands, it has been proposed that insulin acts as a factor that reverses GD-increased NO synthesis and L-arginine transport to values in cells from normal pregnancies. This insulin dual effect can be explained for a differential expression of IR-A and IR-B in normal and GD pregnancies. Insulin effects are dependet on activation of ARs in several cell types, suggesting that adenosine should be act as an isoform insulin receptor activity regulator. Thus, regarding the GD association with increased hCAT-1 expression and activity, there are several not still answered, for example, how is insulin decreasing hCAT-1 activity and expression?, and is adenosine a modulator of the expression and associated signaling of the isoforms of insulin receptors in GD?. Answering these (and other) questions will help us understand insulin mechanisms, opening the possibility to study potential treatment for insulin resistence pathologies including GD.

Acknowledgements

We are thankfull to the personnel at the Hospital Clínico Pontificia Universidad Católica de Chile labour ward for their support in the supply of placentas.This research was supported by Fondo Nacional de Desarrollo Científico y Tecnológico (FONDECYT 1110977, 11110059, 3130583), Programa de Investigación Interdisciplinario (PIA) from Comisión Nacional de Investigación en Ciencia y Tecnología (CONICYT, Anillos ACT-73) (Chile) and CONICYT Ayuda de Tesis (CONICYT AT-24120944). EG-G and PA hold CONICYT-PhD (Chile) fellowships. FP was the recipient of a postdoctoral position (CONICYT PIA Anillos ACT-73 post-doctoral research associate at CMPL, Pontificia Universidad Católica de Chile (PUC)). PA is the recipient of a Faculty of Medicine (PUC) PhD fellowship.

Author details

Enrique Guzmán-Gutiérrez*, Pablo Arroyo, Fabián Pardo, Andrea Leiva and Luis Sobrevia

*Address all correspondence to: elguzman@uc.cl, sobrevia@med.puc.cl

Cellular and Molecular Physiology Laboratory (CMPL), Division of Obstetrics and Gynaecology, School of Medicine, Faculty of Medicine, Pontificia Universidad Católica de Chile, Santiago, Chile

References

[1] Albritton LM, Bowcock AM, Eddy RL, Morton CC, Tseng L, et al. The human cationic amino acid transporter (ATRC1): physical and genetic mapping to 13q12-q14. Genomics 12: 430-434.

[2] Aljada A, Ghanim H, Saadeh R, Dandona P. (2001) Insulin inhibits NFkappaB and MCP-1 expression in human aortic endothelial cells. J Clin Endocrinol Metab 86: 450-453.

[3] American diabetes association (ADA).(2004) Gestational diabetes mellitus. Diabetes Care 27: S88-S90.

[4] American Diabetes Association.(2012) Diagnosis and Classification of Diabetes Mellitus. Diabetes care 35: S64-S71.

[5] Arancibia-Garavilla Y, Toledo F, Casanello P, Sobrevia L. (2003) Nitric oxide synthesis requires activity of the cationic and neutral amino acid transport system y+L in human umbilical vein endothelium. Exp Physiol 88: 699-710.

[6] Ardiansyah HS, Yumi S, Takuya K, Michio K. (2010) Anti-metabolic syndrome effects of adenosine ingestion in stroke-prone spontaneously hypertensive rats fed a high-fat diet. Br J Nutr 104: 48-55.

[7] Aulak KS, Liu J, Wu J, Hyatt SL, Puppi M, et al. (1996) Molecular sites of regulation of expression of the rat cationic amino acid transporter gene. J Biol Chem 271: 29799-29806.

[8] Aulak KS, Mishra R, Zhou L, Hyatt SL, de Jonge W, et al. (1999) Post-transcriptional regulation of the arginine transporter Cat-1 by amino acid availability. J Biol Chem 271: 30424-30432.

[9] Baldwin AS Jr. (1996) The NF-kappa B and I kappa B proteins: new discoveries and insights. Annu Rev Immunol 14: 649-683.

[10] Baldwin SA, Beal PR, Yao SY, King AE, Cass CE, et al. (2004) The equilibrative nucleoside transporter family, SLC29. Pflugers Arch 447: 735-743.

[11] Banfi C, Eriksson P, Giandomenico G, Mussoni L, Sironi L, et al. (2001) Transcriptional regulation of plasminogen activator inhibitor type 1 gene by insulin: insights into the signaling pathway. Diabetes 50: 1522-1530.

[12] Barrett HL, Morris J, McElduff A. (2009) Watchful waiting: a management protocol for maternal glycaemia in the peripartum period. Aust N Z J Obstet Gynaecol 49: 162-167.

[13] Bar-Yehuda S, Stemmer SM, Madi L, Castel D, Ochaion A, et al. (2008) The A3 adenosine receptor agonist CF102 induces apoptosis of hepatocellular carcinoma via de-

regulation of the Wnt and NF-kappaB signal transduction pathways. Int J Oncol 33: 287-295.

[14] Becker BF, Kupatt C, Massoudy P, Zahler S. (2000) Reactive oxygen species and nitric oxide in myocardial ischemia and reperfusion. Z Kardiol 89: 88-91.

[15] Belfiore A, Frasca F, Pandini G, Sciacca L, Vigneri R. (2009) Insulin Receptor Isoforms and Insulin Receptor/Insulin-Like Growth Factor Receptor Hybrids in Physiology and Disease. Endocr Rev 30: 586–623.

[16] Bergandi L, Silvagno F, Russo I, Riganti C, Anfossi G, et al. (2003) Insulin stimulates glucose transport via nitric oxide/cyclic GMP pathway in human vascular smooth muscle cells. Arterioscler Thromb Vasc Biol 23: 2215-2221

[17] Berne RM, Knabb RM, Ely SW, Rubio R. (1983) Adenosine in the local regulation of blood flow: a brief overview. Fed Proc 42: 3136-3142.

[18] Biri A, Onan A, Devrim E, Babacan F, Kavutcu M, et al. (2006) Oxidant status in maternal and cord plasma and placental tissue in gestational diabetes. Placenta 27: 327-32.

[19] Brown MA, North L, Hargood J. (1990) Uteroplacental Doppler ultrasound in routine antenatal care. Aust N Z J Obstet Gynaecol 30: 303-307.

[20] Burgdorf C, Richardt D, Kurz T, Seyfarth M, Jain D, et al. (2001) Adenosine inhibits norepinephrine release in the postischemic rat heart: the mechanism of neuronal stunning. Cardiovasc Res 49: 713-720.

[21] Burgdorf C, Schütte F, Kurz T, Dendorfer A, Richardt G. (2005) Adenylyl cyclase-dependent inhibition of myocardial norepinephrine release by presynaptic adenosine A1-receptors. J Cardiovasc Pharmacol 45 :1-3.

[22] Burnstock G, Fredholm BB, North RA, Verkhratsky A. (2010) The birth and postnatal development of purinergic signalling. Acta Physiol 199: 93-147.

[23] Burnstock G. (2006) Vessel tone and remodeling.Nat Med 12:16-17.

[24] Bussolati O, Sala R, Astorri A, Rotoli BM, Dall'Asta V, et al. (1993). Characterization of amino acid transport in human endothelial cells. Am J Physiol 265: C1006-C1014.

[25] Carr CS, Hill RJ, Masamune H, Kennedy SP, Knight DR, et al. (1997) Evidence for a role for both the adenosine A1 and A3 receptors in protection of isolated human atrial muscle against simulated ischaemia. Cardiovasc Res 36: 52-59.

[26] Casanello P, Escudero C, Sobrevia L. (2007) Equilibrative nucleoside (ENTs) and cationic amino acid (CATs) transporters: implications in foetal endothelial dysfunction in human pregnancy diseases. Curr Vasc Pharmacol 5: 69-84.

[27] Casanello P, Sobrevia L. (2002) Intrauterine growth retardation is associated with reduced activity and expression of the cationic amino acid transport systems y+/

hCAT-1 and y+/hCAT-2B and lower activity of nitric oxide synthase in human umbilical vein endothelial cells. Circ Res 91: 127-134.

[28] Ciaraldi TP, Morales AJ, Hickman MG, Odom-Ford R, Olefsky JM, et al. (1997) Cellular insulin resistance in adipocytes from obese polycystic ovary syndrome subjects involves adenosine modulation of insulin sensitivity. J Clin Endocrinol Metab 82: 1421-1425.

[29] Closs EI, Boissel JP, Habermeier A, Rotmann A. (2006) Structure and function of cationic amino acid transporters (CATs). J Membr Biol 213: 67-77.

[30] Colomiere M, Permezel M, Riley C, Desoye G, Lappas M. (2009) Defective insulin signaling in placenta from pregnancies complicated by gestational diabetes mellitus. Eur J Endocrinol 160: 567-578.

[31] Crisostomo PR, Wang Y, Markel TA, Wang M, Lahm T, et al. (2008) Human mesenchymal stem cells stimulated by TNF-alpha, LPS, or hypoxia produce growth factors by an NF kappa B- but not JNK-dependent mechanism. Am J Physiol Cell Physiol 294: C675-C682.

[32] Dandona P, Aljada A, Mohanty P, Ghanim H, Hamouda W, et al. (2001) Insulin inhibits intranuclear nuclear factor kappaB and stimulates IkappaB in mononuclear cells in obese subjects: evidence for an anti-inflammatory effect? J Clin Endocrinol Metab 86: 3257-3265.

[33] Danialou G, Vicaut E, Sambe A, Aubier M, Boczkowski J. (1997) Predominant role of A1 adenosine receptors in mediating adenosine induced vasodilatation of rat diaphragmatic arterioles: involvement of nitric oxide and the ATP-dependent K+ channels. Br J Pharmacol 121: 1355-1363.

[34] De Vriese AS, Verbeuren TJ, Van de Voorde J, Lameire NH, Vanhoutte PM. (2000) Endothelial dysfunction in diabetes. Br J Pharmacol 130: 963-974.

[35] Derave W, Hespel P. (1999) Role of adenosine in regulating glucose uptake during contractions and hypoxia in rat skeletal muscle. J Physiol 515: 255-263.

[36] Desoye G, and Hauguel-de Mouzon S. (2007) The human placenta in gestational diabetes mellitus. The insulin and cytokine network. Diabetes Care 30: S120-S126.

[37] Devés R, Boyd CA. (1998) Transporters for cationic amino acids in animal cells: discovery, structure, and function. Physiol Rev 78: 487-545.

[38] Dhalla AK, Santikul M, Chisholm JW, Belardinelli L, Reaven GM. (2009) Comparison of the antilipolytic effects of an A1 adenosine receptor partial agonist in normal and diabetic rats. Diabetes Obes Metab 11: 95-101.

[39] Dye JF, Vause S, Johnston T, Clark P, Firth JA, et al. (2004) Characterization of cationic amino acid transporters and expression of endothelial nitric oxide synthase in human placental microvascular endothelial cells. FASEB J 18: 125-127.

[40] Ebina Y, Ellis L, Jarnagin K, Edery M, Graf L, et al. (1985) The human insulin receptor cDNA: the structural basis for hormone-activated transmembrane signalling. Cell 40: 747-758.

[41] Edmunds NJ, Marshall JM. (2003) The roles of nitric oxide in dilating proximal and terminal arterioles of skeletal muscle during systemic hypoxia. J Vasc Res 40: 68-76.

[42] Eltzschig HK. (2009) Adenosine: an old drug newly discovered. Anesthesiology 111: 904-915.

[43] Escudero C, Bertoglia P, Hernadez M, Celis C, González M, et al. (2012) Impaired A(2A) adenosine receptor/nitric oxide/VEGF signaling pathway in fetal endothelium during late- and early-onset preeclampsia. Purinergic signaling 10.1007/s11302-012-9341-4 (In Press).

[44] Escudero C, Puebla C, Westermeier F, Sobrevia L. (2009) Potential cell signalling mechanisms involved in differential placental angiogenesis in mild and severe preeclampsia. Curr Vasc Pharmacol 7: 475-485.

[45] Escudero C, Sobrevia L. (2008) A hypothesis for preeclampsia: adenosine and inducible nitric oxide synthase in human placental microvascular endothelium. Placenta 29: 469-483.

[46] Espinal J, Dohm GL, Newsholme EA. (1983) Sensitivity to insulin of glycolysis and glycogen synthesis of isolated soleus-muscle strips from sedentary, exercised and exercise-trained rats. *Biochem J* 212: 453-458.

[47] Farías M, Puebla C, Westermeier F, Jo MJ, Pastor-Anglada M, et al. (2010) Nitric oxide reduces SLC29A1 promoter activity and adenosine transport involving transcription factor complex hCHOP-C/EBPalpha in human umbilical vein endothelial cells from gestational diabetes. Cardiovasc Res 86: 45-54.

[48] Farías M, San Martin R, Puebla C, Pearson JD, Casado JF, et al. (2006) Nitric oxide reduces adenosine transporter ENT1 gene (SLC29A1) promoter activity in human fetal endothelium from gestational diabetes. J Cell Physiol 208: 451-460.

[49] Feoktistov I, Goldstein AE, Ryzhov S, Zeng D, Belardinelli L, et al. (2002) Differential expression of adenosine receptors in human endothelial cells: role of A2B receptors in angiogenic factor regulation. Circ Res 90: 531-538.

[50] Fernandez J, Lopez AB, Wang C, Mishra R, Zhou L, et al. (2003) Transcriptional control of the arginine/lysine transporter, cat-1, by physiological stress. J Biol Chem 278: 50000-50009.

[51] Fernandez P, Jara C, Aguilera V, Caviedes L, Diaz F, et al. (2012) Adenosine A_2A and A_3 receptors are involved in the human endothelial progenitor cells migration. J Cardiovasc Pharmacol 59: 397-404.

[52] Figler RA, Wang G, Srinivasan S, Jung DY, Zhang Z, et al. (2011) Links between insulin resistance, adenosine A2B receptors, and inflammatory markers in mice and humans. Diabetes 60: 669-679.

[53] Figueroa R, Martinez E, Fayngersh RP, Tejani N, Mohazzab-H KM, et al. (2000) Alterations in relaxation to lactate and H(2)O(2) in human placental vessels from gestational diabetic pregnancies. Am J Physiol Heart Circ Physiol 278: H706-H713.

[54] Fishman P, Bar-Yehuda S, Madi L, Rath-Wolfson L, Ochaion A, et al. (2006) The PI3K-NF-kappaB signal transduction pathway is involved in mediating the anti-inflammatory effect of IB-MECA in adjuvant-induced arthritis. Arthritis Res Ther 8:R33.

[55] Flores C, Rojas S, Aguayo C, Parodi J, Mann G, et al. (2003) Rapid stimulation of L-arginine transport by D-glucose involves p42/44(mapk) and nitric oxide in human umbilical vein endothelium. Circ Res 92: 64-72.

[56] Frasca F, Pandini G, Scalia P, Sciacca L, Mineo R, et al. (1999) Insulin receptor isoform A, a newly recognized, high-affinity insulin-like growth factor II receptor in fetal and cancer cells. Mol Cell Biol 19: 3278-3288.

[57] Fredholm BB, Ijzerman AP, Jacobson KA, Klotz KN, Linden J. (2001) Nomenclature and Classification of Adenosine Receptors. Pharmacol Rev 53; 527-552.

[58] Fredholm BB, IJzerman AP, Jacobson KA, Linden J, Müller CE.(2011) International Union of Basic and Clinical Pharmacology. LXXXI. Nomenclature and classification of adenosine receptors--an update. Pharmacol Rev 63: 1-34.

[59] Fredholm BB. (2007) Adenosine, an endogenous distress signal, modulates tissue damage and repair. Cell Death Differ 14: 1315-1323.

[60] Genua M, Pandini G, Cassarino MF, Messina RL, Frasca F. (2009) c-Abl and insulin receptor signalling. Vitam Horm 80: 77-105.

[61] González M, Flores C, Pearson JD, Casanello P, Sobrevia L. (2004) Cell signalling-mediating insulin increase of mRNA expression for cationic amino acid transporters-1 and -2 and membrane hyperpolarization in human umbilical vein endothelial cells. Pflugers Arch 448: 383-394.

[62] González M, Gallardo V, Rodríguez N, Salomón C, Westermeier F, et al. (2011a) Insulin-stimulated L-arginine transport requires SLC7A1 gene expression and is associated with human umbilical vein relaxation. J Cell Physiol 226: 2916-2924.

[63] González M, Muñoz E, Puebla C, Guzmán-Gutiérrez E, Cifuentes F, et al. (2011b) Maternal and fetal metabolic dysfunction in pregnancy diseases associated with vascular oxidative and nitrative stress. In: *The Molecular Basis for Origin of Fetal Congenital Abnormalities and Maternal Health: An overview of Association with Oxidative Stress.*Eds. BM Matata, M Elahi. Ed. Bentham, USA. Chapter 8, pp 98-115.

[64] Green A. (1987) Adenosine receptor down-regulation and insulin resistance following prolonged incubation of adipocytes with an A1 adenosine receptor agonist. J Biol Chem 262: 15702-15707.

[65] Greene MF, Solomon CG. (2005) Gestational diabetes mellitus -- time to treat. N Engl J Med 352: 2544-2546.

[66] Grillo MA, Lanza A, Colombatto S. (2008) Transport of amino acids through the placenta and their role. Amino Acids 34: 517-523.

[67] Grimm S, Baeuerle PA. (1993) The inducible transcription factor NF-kappa B: structure-function relationship of its protein subunits. Biochem J 290: 297-308.

[68] Guzmán-Gutiérrez E, Westermeier F, Salomón C, González M, Pardo F, et al. (2012a) Insulin-increased L-arginine transport requires A(2A) adenosine receptors activation in human umbilical vein endothelium. PLoS One 7: e41705.

[69] Guzmán-Gutiérrez E, Salomón C, Pardo A, Leiva A, Sobrevia L. (2012b) Insulin reverses gestational diabetes-increased L-arginine transport involving A_1 and A_2A adenosine receptors activation in HUVEC. J Mol Cell Cardiol 53: S15-S16 (Abstract).

[70] Hammermann R, Brunn G, Racké K. (2001) Analysis of the genomic organization of the human cationic amino acid transporters CAT-1, CAT-2 and CAT-4. Amino Acids 21: 211-219.

[71] Han DH, Hansen PA, Nolte LA, Holloszy JO. (1998) Removal of adenosine decreases the responsiveness of muscle glucose transport to insulin and contractions. Diabetes 47: 1671-1675.

[72] Hatzoglou M, Fernandez J, Yaman I, Closs E. (2004) Regulation of cationic amino acid transport: the story of the CAT-1 transporter. Annu Rev Nutr 24: 377-399.

[73] Hiden U, Lang I, Ghaffari-Tabrizi N, Gauster M, Lang U, et al. (2009) Insulin action on the human placental endothelium in normal and diabetic pregnancy. Curr Vasc Pharmacol 7: 460-466.

[74] Horovitz-Fried M, Brutman-Barazani T, Kesten D, Sampson SR. (2008) Insulin increases nuclear protein kinase Cdelta in L6 skeletal muscle cells. Endocrinology 149: 1718-1727.

[75] Huang CJ, Tsai PS, Yang CH, Su TH, Stevens BR, et al. (2004) Pulmonary transcription of CAT-2 and CAT-2B but not CAT-1 and CAT-2A were upregulated in hemorrhagic shock rats. Resuscitation 63: 203-212.

[76] Irie K, Tsukahara F, Fujii E, Uchida Y, Yoshioka T, He WR, et al. (1997) Cationic amino acid transporter-2 mRNA induction by tumor necrosis factor-alpha in vascular endothelial cells. Eur J Pharmacol 339: 289-293.

[77] Jo M, Krause B, Casanello P, Sobrevia L. (2009) Differential reactivity to insulin in human umbilical and chorionic vessels from normal and gestational diabetic pregnancies. DOHaD 1:S307 (abstract).

[78] Johansson GS, Arnqvist HJ.(2006) Insulin and IGF-I action on insulin receptors, IGF-I receptors, and hybrid insulin/IGF-I receptors in vascular smooth muscle cells.Am J Physiol Endocrinol Metab 291: 1124-1130.

[79] Joost HG, Steinfelder HJ. (1982) Modulation of insulin sensitivity by adenosine. Effects on glucose transport, lipid synthesis, and insulin receptors of the adipocyte. Mol Pharmacol 22: 614-618.

[80] Jung YD, Fan F, McConkey DJ, Jean ME, Liu W, et al. (2002) Role of P38 MAPK, AP-1, and NF-kappaB in interleukin-1beta-induced IL-8 expression in human vascular smooth muscle cells. Cytokine 18:206-213.

[81] Ke RH, Xiong J, Liu Y, Ye ZR. (2009) Adenosine A2a receptor induced gliosis via Akt/NF-kappaB pathway in vitro. Neurosci Res 65: 280-285.

[82] Kim JA, Montagnani M, Koh KK, Quon MJ. (2006) Reciprocal relationships between insulin resistance and endothelial dysfunction: molecular and pathophysiological mechanisms. Circulation 113: 1888-1904.

[83] Klinger M, Freissmuth M, Nanoff C. (2002) Adenosine receptors: G protein-mediated signalling and the role of accessory proteins. Cell Signal 2: 99-108.

[84] Kolnes AJ, Ingvaldsen A, Bolling A, Stuenaes JT, Kreft M, et al. (2010) Caffeine and theophylline block insulin-stimulated glucose uptake and PKB phosphorylation in rat skeletal muscles. Acta Physiol (Oxf) 200: 65-74.

[85] Kristensen C, Wiberg FC, Schäffer L, Andersen AS. (1998) Expression and characterization of a 70-kDa fragment of the insulin receptor that binds insulin. Minimizing ligand binding domain of the insulin receptor. J Biol Chem 273: 17780-17786.

[86] Kuzuya T, Matsuda A. (1997) Classification of diabetes on the basis of etiologies versus degree of insulin deficiency. Diabetes Care 20: 219-220.

[87] Laine H, Nuutila P, Luotolahti M, Meyer C, Elomaa T, et al. (2000) Insulin-induced increment of coronary flow reserve is not abolished by dexamethasone in healthy young men. J Clin Endocrinol Metab 85: 1868-1873.

[88] Laine H, Sundell J, Nuutila P, Raitakari OT, Luotolahti M, et al. (2004) Insulin induced increase in coronary flow reserve is abolished by dexamethasone in young men with uncomplicated type 1 diabetes. Heart 90: 270-276.

[89] Lam JK, Matsubara S, Mihara K, Zheng XL, Mooradian AD, et al. (2003) Insulin induction of apolipoprotein AI, role of Sp1. Biochemistry 42: 2680-2690.

[90] Latham AM, Bruns AF, Kankanala J, Johnson AP, Fishwick CW, et al. (2012) Indolinones and anilinophthalazines differentially target VEGF-A- and basic fibroblast

growth factor-mediated responses in primary human endothelial cells. Br J Pharmacol 165: 245-259.

[91] Leibovich SJ, Chen JF, Pinhal-Enfield G, Belem PC, Elson G, et al. (2002) Synergistic up-regulation of vascular endothelial growth factor expression in murine macrophages by adenosine A(2A) receptor agonists and endotoxin. Am J Pathol 160: 2231-2244.

[92] Leiva A, Pardo F, Ramírez MA, Farías M, Casanello P, et al. (2011) Fetoplacental vascular endothelial dysfunction as an early phenomenon in the programming of human adult diseases in subjects born from gestational diabetes mellitus or obesity in pregnancy. Exp Diabetes Res 2011:349286.

[93] Lindsay RS, Westgate JA, Beattie J, Pattison NS, Gamble G, et al. (2007) Inverse changes in fetal insulin-like growth factor (IGF)-1 and IGF binding protein-1 in association with higher birth weight in maternal diabetes. Clin Endocrinol 66: 322-328.

[94] Liu SH, Shan LM, Wang H. (2002) Pharmacological characteristics of novel putative purinoceptors in vascular endothelium. Cell Biol Int 26:963-969.

[95] Madi L, Cohen S, Ochayin A, Bar-Yehuda S, Barer F, et al. (2007) Overexpression of A3 adenosine receptor in peripheral blood mononuclear cells in rheumatoid arthritis: involvement of nuclear factor-kappaB in mediating receptor level. J Rheumatol 34: 20-26.

[96] Maguire MH, Szabó I, Valkó IE, Finley BE, Bennett TL. (1998) Simultaneous measurement of adenosine and hypoxanthine in human umbilical cord plasma using reversed-phase high-performance liquid chromatography with photodiode-array detection and on-line validation of peak purity.J Chromatogr B Biomed Sci Appl 707: 33-41.

[97] Marzioni D, Tamagnone L, Capparuccia L, Marchini C, Amici A, et al. (2004) Restricted innervation of uterus and placenta during pregnancy: evidence for a role of the repelling signal Semaphorin 3A. Dev Dyn 231: 839-848.

[98] Mate A, Vázquez CM, Leiva A, Sobrevía L. (2012) New therapeutic approaches to treating hypertension in pregnancy. Drug Discov Today 17: 1307-1315.

[99] Metzger BE, Buchanan TA, Coustan DR, de Leiva A, Dunger DB, et al. (2007) Summary and recommendations of the Fifth International Workshop-Conference on Gestational Diabetes Mellitus. Diabetes Care 30: S251-S260.

[100] Metzger BE, Coustan DR. (1998) Summary and recommendations of the Fourth International Workshop-Conference on Gestational Diabetes Mellitus. The Organizing Committee. Diabetes Care 21: B161-B167.

[101] Mohan S, Hamuro M, Koyoma K, Sorescu GP, Jo H, et al. (2003) High glucose induced NF-kappaB DNA-binding activity in HAEC is maintained under low shear

stress but inhibited under high shear stress: role of nitric oxide. Atherosclerosis 171: 225-234.

[102] Moller DE, Yokota A, White MF, Pazianos AG, Flier JS. (1989) A naturally occurring mutation of insulin receptor alanine 1134 impairs tyrosine kinase function and is associated with dominantly inherited insulin resistance. J Biol Chem 265: 14979–14985.

[103] Montecinos VP, Aguayo C, Flores C, Wyatt AW, Pearson JD, et al. (2000) Regulation of adenosine transport by D-glucose in human fetal endothelial cells: involvement of nitric oxide, protein kinase C and mitogen-activated protein kinase. J Physiol 529: 777-790.

[104] Montesinos MC, Shaw JP, Yee H, Shamamian P, Cronstein BN. (2004). Adenosine A(2A) receptor activation promotes wound neovascularization by stimulating angiogenesis and vasculogenesis. Am J Pathol 164: 1887-1892.

[105] Morello S, Sorrentino R, Porta A, Forte G, Popolo A, et al. (2009) Cl-IB-MECA enhances TRAIL-induced apoptosis via the modulation of NF-kappaB signalling pathway in thyroid cancer cells. J Cell Physiol 221: 378-386.

[106] Morisset AS, St-Yves A, Veillette J, Weisnagel SJ, Tchernof A, et al. (2010) Prevention of gestational diabetes mellitus: a review of studies on weight management. Diabetes Metab Res Rev 26: 17-25.

[107] Mosthaf L, Vogt B, Häring HU, Ullrich A. (1991) Altered expression of insulin receptor types A and B in the skeletal muscle of non-insulin-dependent diabetes mellitus patients. Proc Natl Acad Sci U S A 88: 4728-4730.

[108] Mounier C, Posner BI. (2006) Transcriptional regulation by insulin: from the receptor to the gene. Can J Physiol Pharmacol 84: 713-724.

[109] Mundell S, Kelly E. (2010) Adenosine receptor desensitization and trafficking. Biochim Biophys Acta 1808: 1319-1328.

[110] Muniyappa R, Montagnani M, Koh KK, Quon MJ. (2007) Cardiovascular actions of insulin. Endocr Rev 28: 463-491.

[111] Muñoz G, San Martín R, Farías M, Cea L, Casanello P, et al. (2006) Insulin restores glucose–inhibition of adenosine transport by increasing the expression and activity of the equilibrative nucleoside transporter 2 in human umbilical vein endothelium. J Cell Physiol 209: 826-835.

[112] Murao K, Wada Y, Nakamura T, Taylor AH, Mooradian AD, et al. (1998) Effects of glucose and insulin on rat apolipoprotein A-I gene expression. J Biol Chem 273: 18959-18965.

[113] Nakao S, Ogtata Y, Shimizu E, Yamazaki M, Furuyama S, et al. (2002) Tumor necrosis factor alpha (TNF-alpha)-induced prostaglandin E2 release is mediated by the

activation of cyclooxygenase-2 (COX-2) transcription via NFkappaB in human gingival fibroblasts. Mol Cell Biochem 238: 11-18.

[114] Németh ZH, Bleich D, Csóka B, Pacher P, Mabley JG, et al. (2007) Adenosine receptor activation ameliorates type 1 diabetes. FASEB J 21: 2379-2388.

[115] Nitert MD, Chisalita SI, Olsson K, Bornfeldt KE, Arnqvist HJ. (2005) IGF-I/insulin hybrid receptors in human endothelial cells. Mol Cell Endocrinol 229: 31-37.

[116] Nold JL, Georgieff MK. (2004) Infants of diabetic mothers. Pediatr Clin North Am 51: 619-637.

[117] Norgren S, Li LS, Luthman H. (1994) Regulation of human insulin receptor RNA splicing in HepG2 cells: effects of glucocorticoid and low glucose concentration. Biochem Biophys Res Commun 199: 277-284.

[118] Olanrewaju HA, Mustafa SJ. (2000). Adenosine A(2A) and A(2B) receptors mediated nitric oxide production in coronary artery endothelial cells. Gen Pharmacol 35: 171-177.

[119] Olsson RA, Pearson JD. (1990) Cardiovascular purinoceptors. Physiol Rev 70: 761-845.

[120] Pandini G, Frasca F, Mineo R, Sciacca L, Vigneri R, et al. (2002) Insulin/insulin-like growth factor I hybrid receptors have different biological characteristics depending on the insulin receptor isoform involved. J Biol Chem 277: 39684-39695.

[121] Pandolfi A, Di Pietro N. (2010) High glucose, nitric oxide, and adenosine: a vicious circle in chronic hyperglycaemia? Cardiovasc Res 86: 9-11.

[122] Pardo F, Arroyo P, Salomón C, Westermeier F, Guzmán-Gutiérrez E, et al. (2012) Gestational Diabetes Mellitus and the Role of Adenosine in the Human Placental Endothelium and Central Nervous System. J Diabetes Metab S2:010. doi: 10.4172/2155-6156.S2-010

[123] Pawelczyk T, Sakowicz-Burkiewicz M, Kocbuch K, Szutowicz A. (2005) Differential effect of insulin and elevated glucose level on adenosine handling in rat T lymphocytes. J Cell Biochem 96: 1296-1310.

[124] Phillips DI. (1998) Birth weight and the future development of diabetes.A review of the evidence. Diabetes Care 21: 150-155.

[125] Pietryga M, Brazert J, Wender-Ozegowska E, Dubiel M, Gudmundsson S. (2006) Placental Doppler velocimetry in gestational diabetes mellitus. J Perinat Med 34: 108-110.

[126] Puebla C, Farías M, González M, Vecchiola A, Aguayo C, et al. (2008) High D-glucose reduces SLC29A1 promoter activity and adenosine transport involving specific protein 1 in human umbilical vein endothelium. J Cell Physiol 215: 645-656.

http://dx.doi.org/10.5772/55627

[127] Ray CJ, Marshall JM. (2006) The cellular mechanisms by which adenosine evokes release of nitric oxide from rat aortic endothelium. J Physiol 570: 85-96.

[128] Ribé D, Sawbridge D, Thakur S, Hussey M, Ledent C, et al. (2008) Adenosine A2A receptor signaling regulation of cardiac NADPH oxidase activity. Free Radic Biol Med 44: 1433-1442.

[129] Sala R, Rotoli BM, Colla E, Visigalli R, Parolari A, et al. (2002) Two-way arginine transport in human endothelial cells: TNF-alpha stimulation is restricted to system y(+). Am J Physiol Cell Physiol 282: C134-C143.

[130] Salomón C, Westermeier F, Puebla C, Arroyo P, Guzmán-Gutiérrez E, et al. (2012) Gestational diabetes reduces adenosine transport in human placental microvascular endothelium, an effect reversed by insulin. PLoS One 7: e40578.

[131] Samson SL, Wong NC. (2002) Role of Sp1 in insulin regulation of gene expression. J Mol Endocrinol 29: 265-279.

[132] San Martin R, Sobrevia L. (2006) Gestational diabetes and the adenosine/L-arginine/nitric oxide (ALANO) pathway in human umbilical vein endothelium. Placenta 27: 1-10.

[133] Sands WA, Martin AF, Strong EW, Palmer TM. (2004) Specific inhibition of nuclear factor-kappaB-dependent inflammatory responses by cell type-specific mechanisms upon A2A adenosine receptor gene transfer. Mol Pharmacol 66: 1147-1159.

[134] Savkur R, Philips V, Cooper H. (2001) Aberrant regulation of insulin receptor alternative splicing is associated with insulin resistance in myotonic dystrophy. Nat Genet 29: 40-47.

[135] Schulte G, Fredholm BB. (2003) The G(s)-coupled adenosine A (2B) receptor recruits divergent pathways to regulate ERK1/2 and p38. Exp Cell Res 290: 168-176.

[136] Sciacca L, Cassarino MF, Genua M, Pandini G, Le Moli R, et al. (2010) Insulin analogues differently activate insulin receptor isoforms and post-receptor signalling. Diabetologia 53: 1743-1753.

[137] Sciacca L, Prisco M, Wu A, Belfiore A, Vigneri R, et al. (2003) Signaling differences from the A and B isoforms of the insulin receptor (IR) in 32D cells in the presence or absence of IR substrate-1. Endocrinology 144: 2650-2658.

[138] Seino S, Seino M, Nishi S, Bell GI. (1989) Structure of the human insulin receptor gene and characterization of its promoter. Proc Natl Acad Sci U S A 86: 114-118.

[139] Sen S, Talukdar I, Liu Y, Tam J, Reddy S, et al. (2010) Muscleblind-like 1 (Mbnl1) promotes insulin receptor exon 11 inclusion via binding to a downstream evolutionarily conserved intronic enhancer. J Biol Chem 285: 25426-25437.

[140] Sesti G, Federici M, Lauro D, Sbraccia P, Lauro R. (2001) Molecular mechanism of insulin resistance in type 2 diabetes mellitus: role of the insulin receptor variant forms. Diabetes Metab Res Rev 17: 363-373.

[141] Shen J, Halenda SP, Sturek M, Wilden PA. (2005) Cell-signaling evidence for adenosine stimulation of coronary smooth muscle proliferation via the A1 adenosine receptor. Circ Res 97: 574-582.

[142] Shepherd PR. (2004) Secrets of insulin and IGF-1 regulation of insulin secretion revealed. Biochem J 377: e1-e2.

[143] Sheu ML, Chao KF, Sung YJ, Lin WW, Lin-Shiau SY, et al. (2005) Activation of phosphoinositide 3-kinase in response to inflammation and nitric oxide leads to the upregulation of cyclooxygenase-2 expression and subsequent cell proliferation in mesangial cells. Cell Signal 17: 975-984.

[144] Shryock JC, Snowdy S, Baraldi PG, Cacciari B, Spalluto G, et al. (1998) A2A-adenosine receptor reserve for coronary vasodilation. Circulation 98: 711-718.

[145] Simmons WW, Closs EI, Cunningham JM, Smith TW, Kelly RA. (1996) Cytokines and insulin induce cationic amino acid transporter (CAT) expression in cardiac myocytes. Regulation of L-arginine transport and no production by CAT-1, CAT-2A, and CAT-2B.J Biol Chem 271: 11694-702.

[146] Sobrevia L, Abarzúa F, Nien JK, Salomón C, Westermeier F, et al. (2011) Review: Differential placental macrovascular and microvascular endothelial dysfunction in gestational diabetes. Placenta 32: S159-S164.

[147] Sobrevia L, Cesare P, Yudilevich DL, Mann GE. (1995) Diabetes-induced activation of system y+ and nitric oxide synthase in human endothelial cells: association with membrane hyperpolarization. J Physiol 489:183-192.

[148] Sobrevia L, Mann GE. (1997) Dysfunction of the endothelial L-arginine-nitric oxide signalling pathway in diabetes and hyperglycaemia.Exp Physiol 82: 1-30.

[149] Sobrevia L, Puebla C, Farías M, Casanello P. (2009). Role of equilibrative nucleoside transporters in fetal endothelial dysfunction in gestational diabetes. In: *Membrane Transporters and Receptors in Disease.* Eds. L Sobrevia, P Casanello. Ed. Research Signpost, India. Chapter 1, pp 1-25.

[150] Sobrevia L, Yudilevich DL, Mann GE. (1998) Elevated D-glucose induces insulin insensitivity in human umbilical endothelial cells isolated from gestational diabetic pregnancies. J Physiol 506: 219-230.

[151] Sobrevia L. González M. (2009) A Role for insulin on L-arginine transport in fetal endothelial dysfunction in hyperglycaemia. Curr Vasc Pharmacol 7: 467-474.

[152] Solomon SS, Majumdar G, Martinez-Hernandez A, Raghow R. (2008) A critical role of Sp1 transcription factor in regulating gene expression in response to insulin and other hormones. Life Sci 83: 305-312.

[153] Sonne MP, Højbjerre L, Alibegovic AC, Vaag A, Stallknecht B, et al. (2010) Diminished insulin-mediated forearm blood flow and muscle glucose uptake in young men with low birth weight. J Vasc Res 47: 139-147.

[154] Srinivasan M, Herrero P, McGill JB, Bennik J, Heere B, et al. (2005) The Effects of Plasma Insulin and Glucose on Myocardial Blood Flow in Patients With Type 1 Diabetes Mellitus. J Am Coll Cardiol 46: 42-48.

[155] Steinberg HO, Baron AD. (2002) Vascular function, insulin resistance and fatty acids. Diabetologia 45: 623-634.

[156] Sullivan GW, Lee DD, Ross WG, DiVietro JA, Lappas CM, et al. (2004) Activation of A2A adenosine receptors inhibits expression of alpha 4/beta 1 integrin (very late antigen-4) on stimulated human neutrophils. J Leukoc Biol 75: 127-134.

[157] Sundell J, Knuuti J. (2003) Insulin and myocardial blood flow. Cardiovasc Res 57: 312-319.

[158] Sundell J, Laine H, Nuutila P, Rönnemaa T, Luotolahti M, et al. (2002) The effects of insulin and short-term hyperglycaemia on myocardial blood flow in young men with uncomplicated Type I diabetes. Diabetologia 45: 775-782.

[159] Tchirikov M, Rybakowski C, Hüneke B, Schoder V, Schröder HJ. (2002) Umbilical vein blood volume flow rate and umbilical artery pulsatility as 'venous-arterial index' in the prediction of neonatal compromise. Ultrasound Obstet Gynecol 20: 580-585.

[160] Thakur S, Du J, Hourani S, Ledent C, Li JM. (2010) Inactivation of adenosine A2A receptor attenuates basal and angiotensin II-induced ROS production by Nox2 in endothelial cells. J Biol Chem 285: 40104-40113.

[161] Thorsøe KS, Schlein M, Steensgaard DB, Brandt J, Schluckebier G, et al. (2010) Kinetic evidence for the sequential association of insulin binding sites 1 and 2 to the insulin receptor and the influence of receptor isoform. Biochemistry 49: 6234-6246.

[162] Timmerman KL, Lee JL, Dreyer HC, Dhanani S, Glynn EL, et al. (2010) Insulin stimulates human skeletal muscle protein synthesis via an indirect mechanism involving endothelial-dependent vasodilation and mammalian target of rapamycin complex 1 signaling. J Clin Endocrinol Metab 95: 3848-3857.

[163] Tong BC, Barbul A. (2004) Cellular and physiological effects of arginine. Mini Rev Med Chem 4: 823-832.

[164] Töpfer M, Burbiel CE, Müller CE, Knittel J, Verspohl EJ. (2008) Modulation of insulin release by adenosine A1 receptor agonists and antagonists in INS-1 cells: the possible contribution of 86Rb+ efflux and 45Ca2+ uptake. Cell Biochem Funct 26: 833-843.

[165] Tsai PS, Chen CC, Tsai PS, Yang LC, Huang WY, et al. (2006) Heme oxygenase 1, nuclear factor E2-related factor 2, and nuclear factor kappaB are involved in hemin inhibition of type 2 cationic amino acid transporter expression and L-Arginine transport in stimulated macrophages. Anesthesiology 105: 1201-1210.

[166] Ullrich A, Bell JR, Chen EY, Herrera R, Petruzzelli LM, et al. (1985) Human insulin receptor and its relationship to the tyrosine kinase family of oncogenes. Nature 313: 756-761.

[167] Vásquez G, Sanhueza F, Vásquez R, González M, San Martín R, et al. (2004) Role of adenosine transport in gestational diabetes-induced L-arginine transport and nitric oxide synthesis in human umbilical vein endothelium.J Physiol 560: 111-122.

[168] Vásquez R, Farías M, Vega JL, Martin RS, Vecchiola A, et al. (2007) D-glucose stimulation of L-arginine transport and nitric oxide synthesis results from activation of mitogen-activated protein kinases p42/44 and Smad2 requiring functional type II TGF-beta receptors in human umbilical vein endothelium. J Cell Physiol 212: 626-632.

[169] Vergauwen L, Hespel P, Richter EA. (1994) Adenosine receptors mediate synergistic stimulation of glucose uptake and transport by insulin and by contractions in rat skeletal muscle. J Clin Invest 93: 974-981.

[170] Verrey F, Closs EI, Wagner CA, Palacin M, Endou H, et al. (2004) CATs and HATs: the SLC7 family of amino acid transporters. Pflugers Arch 447: 532-542.

[171] Vina-Vilaseca A, Bender-Sigel J, Sorkina T, Closs EI, Sorkin A. (2011) Protein kinase C-dependent ubiquitination and clathrin-mediated endocytosis of the cationic amino acid transporter CAT-1. J Biol Chem 286: 8697-8706.

[172] Visigalli R, Barilli A, Bussolati O, Sala R, Gazzola GC, et al. (2007) Rapamycin stimulates arginine influx through CAT2 transporters in human endothelial cells. Biochim Biophys Acta 1768: 1479-87.

[173] von Mandach U, Lauth D, Huch R. (2003) Maternal and fetal nitric oxide production in normal and abnormal pregnancy. J Matern Fetal Neonatal Med 13: 22-27.

[174] Webster JM, Heseltine L, Taylor R. (1996) In vitro effect of adenosine agonist GR79236 on the insulin sensitivity of glucose utilisation in rat soleus and human rectus abdominus muscle. Biochim Biophys Acta 1316: 109-113.

[175] Westermeier F, Puebla C, Vega JL, Farías M, Escudero C, et al. (2009)Equilibrative Nucleoside Transporters in Fetal Endothelial Dysfunction in Diabetes Mellitus and Hyperglycaemia. Curr Vasc Pharmacol 7:435-449.

[176] Westermeier F, Salomón C, González M, Puebla C, Guzmán-Gutiérrez E, et al. (2011) Insulin restores gestational diabetes mellitus-reduced adenosine transport involving

differential expression of insulin receptor isoforms in human umbilical vein endothelium. Diabetes 60: 1677-1687.

[177] Westgate JA, Lindsay RS, Beattie J, Pattison NS, Gamble G, et al. (2006) Hyperinsulinemia in cord blood in mothers with type 2 diabetes and gestational diabetes mellitus in New Zealand. Diabetes Care 29: 1345-1350.

[178] Wierstra I. (2008) Sp1: emerging roles--beyond constitutive activation of TATA-less housekeeping genes. Biochem Biophys Res Commun 372: 1-13.

[179] Wu G. (2009) Amino acid: metabolism, function, and nutrition. Amino acid 37: 1-17.

[180] Wyatt AW, Steinert JR, Wheeler-Jones CPD, Morgan AJ, Sugden D, et al. (2002) Early activation of the p42/p44 MAPK pathway mediates adenosine-induced nitric oxide production in human endothelial cells: a novel calcium insensitive mechanism. FASEB J 16:1584-1594.

[181] Yan X, Zhu MJ, Xu W, Tong JF, Ford SP, et al. (2010) Up-regulation of Toll-like receptor 4/nuclear factor-kappaB signaling is associated with enhanced adipogenesis and insulin resistance in fetal skeletal muscle of obese sheep at late gestation. Endocrinology 151: 380-387.

[182] Youngren JF. (2007) Regulation of insulin receptor function.Cell. Mol. Life Sci 64: 873-891.

[183] Zeng G, Quon MJ. (1996) Insulin-stimulated production of nitric oxide is inhibited by wortmannin. Direct measurement in vascular endothelial cells. J Clin Invest 98: 894-898.

[184] Zhang WF, Hu DH, Xu CF, Lü GF, Dong ML, et al. (2010) Inhibitory effect of insulin on nuclear factor-kappa B nuclear translocation of vascular endothelial cells induced by burn serum. Zhonghua Shao Shang Za Zhi 26: 175-179.

[185] Zhang WZ, Venardos K, Finch S, Kaye DM. (2008) Detrimental effect of oxidized LDL on endothelial arginine metabolism and transportation. Int J Biochem Cell Biol 40: 920-928.

Chapter 5

Pro-Inflammatory Cytokines, Lipid Metabolism and Inflammation in Gestational Diabetes Mellitus as Cause of Insulin Resistance

Alexander E. Omu

Additional information is available at the end of the chapter

http://dx.doi.org/10.5772/55634

1. Introduction

Gestational diabetes mellitus (GDM) is a glucose intolerance of varying severity with onset or first recognition, during pregnancy that complicates 2–4% of pregnancies (Ben-Haroush et al 2004, American Diabetes Association 2005, NICE Guidelines 2008). Both patients with GDM, and their offspring, have greater risk of developing type 2 diabetes later in life (Damn 1998). There is a close relationship between GDM and prediabetes state in addition to the risk of future deterioration in insulin resistance and ultimate development of overt type 2 diabetes mellitus (Kjos et al 1999). Diabetes in pregnancy is increasing and therefore it is important to raise awareness of the associated health risks to the mother, the growing fetus, and the future child. Perinatal mortality and morbidity is increased in diabetic pregnancies through increased stillbirths and congenital malformation rates (Canadian Diabetes association 2003, HAPO 2008, RCOG SAC 2011). These are mainly the result of early fetal exposure to maternal hyperglycaemia. In the mother, pregnancy may lead to worsening or development of diabetic complications such as retinopathy, nephropathy, and hypoglycaemia (Ali and Dornhorst 2011). Although glycaemic control is important in reducing microvascular complications due to diabetes in pregnancy, it has not reduced the rate of congenital anomalies, macrosomia and other adverse outcomes (Canadian Diabetes Association 2003). This may be as a result of our lack of understanding of the epidemiology and pathogenesis of GDM (Omu et al. 2010), especially the role of inflammation, cytokines and lipid metabolism.

1.1. The main objectives of this review are to draw attention to

a. The epidemiology, genetics and immunological basis of GDM

b. Elucidate the effect of lipid metabolism and lipid peroxidation, oxidative stress on antioxidant gene expression and other inflammatory cytokines.

c. Investigate the role of risk factors including obesity and adipokines like adiponectin, leptin and tumor necrosis factor alpha, acute phase proteins like C-reactive protein (C-RP), IL-6 and plasminogen activation inhibitor -1 (PAI-1) and proinflammatory Cytokines and the mechanisms involved in the pathogenesis.

d. Highlight the role of intervention strategy in the prevention of progression of GDM to type 2 Diabetes Mellitus and alteration of Maternal effects of GDM

2. Epidemiology of gestational diabetes mellitus

Gestational diabetes has been recognised as a heterogenous disorder of glucose intolerance (Kjos et al 1999, Metzger et al 2010, and Omu et al 2011). Unfortunately, comparisons of frequencies of GDM among various populations is difficult because, there are differences in screening programmes and diagnostic criteria (Butte 2000, Ben-Haroush et al 2004, Buchanan et al 2007). There is an urgent need to develop and unify appropriate diabetic diagnostic and prevention strategies and address potentially modifiable risk factors such as obesity.

2.1. Diagnostic criteria of gestational diabetes mellitus (GDM)

Historically, the diagnosis of gestational diabetes mellitus (GDM), like diabetes mellitus in general, has been by measuring the fasting plasma glucose level and performing an oral glucose tolerance test (OGGT) with the threshold as shown in Table 1. In 2010, the American Diabetic Association added haemoglobin A1c (Hb A1c) as a diagnostic tool for individual with type 2 diabetes mellitus with a threshold fixed at 6.5 % for diagnosis. It was however, not recommended for use in GDM.

	mg/dl	**mmol/L**
100g glucose load		
Fasting	95	5.3
1 hour	180	10.0
2 hour	155	8.6
3 hour	140	7.8
75 g glucose load		
Fasting	95	5.3
1 hour	180	10.0
2 hour	155	8.6

Table 1. Diagnosis of Gestational Diabetes Mellitus (GDM)

For diagnosis of GDM, 2 values in each diagnostic group must be met or exceeded (ADA 2011).

http://dx.doi.org/10.5772/55634

According to the NICE guidelines No 63 (2008), screening for GDM using fasting plasma glucose, random blood glucose, glucose challenge test and urinalysis for glucose, should not be recommended. Instead a 2 hour 75 g OGTT should be done at 24-28 weeks of gestation.

2.2. Non-genetic factors

Ethnicity, old age, family history, obesity and high fat diet and sedentary lifestyle, represent some important non-genetic identifiable predisposing factors for GDM, and in the absence of risk factors, there is low incidence of GDM. Ethnicity has been proven to be an independent risk factor for GDM (Dooley et al 1991, Weerakiet et al. 2004) which varies in prevalence in direct proportion to the prevalence of Type 2 diabetes in a given population or ethnic group. Women with an early diagnosis of GDM, in the first half of pregnancy, represent a high-risk subgroup, with an increased incidence of obstetric complications, recurrent GDM in subsequent pregnancies, and future development of Type 2 diabetes(Ben-Housah et al 2004, Buchanan et al 2007). There is a strong association between Gestational Diabetes Mellitus and women with diagnosed Polycystic Ovary Syndrome (PCOS) (Weerakiet et al 2004, Lo et al 2006). The prevalence of GDM is increasing worldwide because of the obesity epidemic and the increasing sedentary lifestyle and the attractive high caloric intake and need for insulin for glycaemic control (Bray et al 2003, Hedley et al 2004, Callagher et al 2008, Kulie et al. 2011, WHO 2011).

2.3. Postpartum diabetes mellitus

Gestational Diabetes Mellitus increases the risk of developing Type1 and Type 2 diabetes mellitus. Risk estimates for type 2 Diabetes is 17 to 68 percent within 5-16 years after pregnancy (O'Sullivan 1991, Hanna et al. 2002, Ben-Housah et. al 2004). The risk factors for postpartum diabetes include islet autoantibody positivity, insulin requirement during pregnancy, Obesity (Lauenborg et al 2004) and strong family history.

2.4. Genetics of GDM

GDM is considered to result from interaction between genetic and environmental risk factors. Women with mutations in MODY (Maturity onset diabetes of the young) genes often present with GDM. Genetic predisposition to GDM has been suggested given the occurrence of the disease within family members. GDM is reported to be often present in women with mutation of MODY gene mutations (Lapolla et al 1996, Ferber et al. 1999, Watanabe et al 2007). Candidate susceptibility gene variants have been suggested to increase the risk of GDM. These genes include glucokinase (GCK), HLA antigens, insulin receptor (INSR), insulin-like growth factor-2 (IGF2), insulin gene (INS-VNTR), plasminogen activator inhibitor 1 (PAI-1), potassium inwardly rectifying channel subfamily J, member 11 (KCNJ11), hepatocyte nuclear factor-4a (HNF4A) (Love-Gregory and Permutt 2007). Identification of the possible underlying genetic factors and mechanisms of the pathogenesis may contribute to the individualization of both prevention and treatment of complications for the mother and fetus (Lambrinoudaki et al 2010). Furthermore, it may improve options to prevent GDM and the complications for the mother and child (Shaat and Groop 2007). During pregnancy, pancreatic cells should by necessity, expand and produce more insulin to adapt to the needs of the pregnancy and the growing baby. Hepatic Growth Factor (HGF) which interact with a surface receptor called c-Met. HGF/c-Met pathway signaling, plays a key role in increasing insulin secretion during pregnancy. The mechanisms in the maternal β-cells adaptation during pregnancy include maternal β-cell hyperplasia by lactogens and HGF/c-Met (Ernst et al 2011). Loss of HGF/c-Met Signaling in Pancreatic β-Cells leads to incomplete Maternal β-Cell Adaptation and Gestational Diabetes Mellitus (Demirci et al 2012).

3. Lipid metabolism and gestational diabetes mellitus

3.1. Lipid and lipoproteins

Hyperlipidemia is a common comorbidity among patients with diabetes mellitus (Anger et al 2011, Koukkou et al 2011). A recent study has found an association between cholesterol intake and GDM (Gonzalez-Clemente et al. 2007). In the placenta, expressions of key proteins involved in de novo lipid synthesis are affected by changes in maternal metabolism (hypercholesterolemia and GDM) that may subsequently affect fetal development and result in asymmetric macrosomia. In addition, impaired placental function gives rise to significant increases in LDL, Apo-B-100 and triglyceride in maternal serum with increased levels of fatty acid synthase (FAS) and SREBP-2 expression and inflammatory cytokines (IL-1β and TNF-α) in placenta (Marseille-Trembley et al 2008). This may give rise to trend towards an increased risk of cardiovascular disease (Gonzalez-Clemente et al. 2007).

3.2. Free fatty acids

Free fatty acids (FFA) are the main circulating lipid fuel. FFA released from visceral depot appear to serve as a marker of systemic insulin resistance and associated increases in cardiovascular risk (Sivan et al 1999, Catalano et al 2002, Jensen 2006). This has been attributed to apoptosis of pancreatic beta cells through pathway involving caspase and ceramide as a mechanism underlying FFA induced impairment of beta –cell function (Turpin et al 2006). Hyperglycaemia and elevated FFA may act synergistically in causing damage to beta cells (El-Assaad et al 2003) and decreases ability of insulin to suppress free fatty acids with advancing gestation with GDM (Darmady and Postle 1982). In a recent report, Schaefer and Colleagues (2011) demonstrated higher free fatty acids in the cord blood of those neonates from mothers with gestational diabetes, indicating their enhanced placental transport and/or enhanced lipolysis as a result of decreased insulin responsiveness (Kautzky-Willer et al 2003).

3.3. Effects of lipid peroxidation

The markers of lipid oxidation, especially malondialdehyde (MDA) increased with hyperglycaemia (Davi et al. 2005). Lipid peroxidation is a crucial process generated naturally in the body, mainly by the effect of several reactive oxygen species such as hydroxyl radical, hydrogen peroxide and superoxide. These reactive oxygen species readily attack the polyunsaturated fatty acids of the fatty acid membrane, initiating a self-propagating chain reaction (Hanachi et al. 2009). The destruction of membrane lipids and the end-products of such lipid peroxidation reactions cause cell damage. Enzymatic (catalase, superoxide dismutase) and nonenzymatic (vitamins A and E) natural antioxidant defense mechanisms exist; however, these mechanisms may be overcome, causing lipid peroxidation to take place. Lipid peroxidation has been implicated in disease states such as atherosclerosis, asthma, Parkinson's disease, kidney damage and preeclampsia (Mylonas and Kouretas 1999, Veskoukis et al 2012)

3.4. Effect of lipid metabolism on neonatal outcome

The development of diabetes in pregnancy induces a state of dyslipidemia, characterized by a high triglyceride concentration (Koukkon et al 1996,) and associated with disturbance of fetal development with modification of key features of placental function (Marseille-Tremblay 2008). GDM patients with macrosomic fetuses are associated with higher lipid and lipoprotein concentrations than in control patients (Mersouk et al. 2000).

8-Isoprostane is a product of lipid peroxidation that can be used as a measure of free radical exposure or injury. Periventricular-intraventricular hemorrhage, necrotizing enterocolitis, chronic lung disease and retinopathy of prematurity have been referred to as oxygen radical diseases (ORD) because they are thought to be related to excess oxidant stress relative to antioxidant defenses in premature infants (Weinberger et al 2006). Umbilical cord venous, but not arterial, 8-isoprostane levels are associated with mortality and the development of one or more of the ORD. In a study, serum triglyceride, total cholesterol, and LDL-c concentrations were higher in the SGA neonates than in AGA neonates, whereas high-density lipoprotein cholesterol concentrations were similar, suggesting a limited ability to clear intravenous lipids in SGA infants (Arends et al 2005). These findings are in agreement with many previous studies in adults and children that show that low birth weight was significantly associated with a less favorable lipid profile (Mortaz et al 2001). Hyperinsulinemia is known to enhance hepatic very-low-density lipoprotein synthesis, which may contribute to increased plasma triglycerides and LDL-c levels. Resistance to the action of insulin on lipoprotein lipase in peripheral tissues may also contribute to elevated triglyceride and LDL-c levels. (Barker et al 1993).

3.5. Adipose tissue as an endocrine organ

The discovery of leptin in the mid-1990s has focused attention on the role of proteins secreted by adipose tissue (Wang et al 2004). Leptin has profound effects on appetite and energy balance, and is also involved in the regulation of neuroendocrine and immune function. Sex steroid and glucocorticoid metabolism in adipose tissue have been implicated as a determinant of body fat distribution and cardiovascular risk. Other adipose products, include other adipokines such as adiponectin, proinflammatory cytokines such as TNF-alpha and IL-6, C-Reactive Protein, complement factors (Cipollini et al 1999, Coppack 2001) and components of the coagulation/fibrinolytic cascade like plasminogen activation inhibitor-1 (PAI-1), that may mediate the metabolic and cardiovascular complications associated with obesity and insulin resistance (Ahima and Flier 2000, Hutley and Prins 2005, Jensen 2006).).

4. Immunology of gestational diabetes

Pregnancy represents a distinct immunologic state in the fetus that acts as an allograft to the mother, needing protection against potential rejection. There is some evidence that inflammation and activated innate immunity is associated with the pathogenesis of Type 2 Diabetes (Pickup 2004), but this needs comfirmation, especially in GDM.

4.1. Humoral reactivity in pregnancy

The placental HLA-G proteins facilitate semiallogeneic pregnancy by inhibiting maternal immune responses to foreign (paternal) antigens via their actions on immune cells is now well established, and the postulate that the recombinant counterparts of these proteins may be used as powerful tools for accommodating the fetus and prevent immune rejection (Hunt et. al 2005). Humoral immune-reactivity does not change much during pregnancy, with the exception of lowered immunoglobulin G concentration at late phase, probably explained by placental transport. Regarding cellular immunity, the reduction, elevation, and lack of variation in the number of different lymphocytic populations, have been reported (Mahmoud et al 2005, 2006).

4.2. Autoimmune GDM

Multiple autoimmune disturbances may be manifested during pregnancy (Leiva et al 2008). Ferber and Associates (1999) have demonstrated that women with GDM who have islet autoantibodies at delivery or develop IDDM postpartum have HLA alleles typical of late-onset type 1 diabetes, and that both HLA typing and islet antibodies can therefore predict the development of postpartum IDDM. Freinkel et al. (1986) first proposed what may be defined as autoimmune GDM; that GDM entails genotypic and phenotypic diversity which may include patients with slowly evolving type 1 diabetes (Mauricio and Leiva 2001, Lapolla et al 2009). There is current consensus that autoimmune GDM is a heterogeneous condition that accounts for 10% of all Caucasian women diagnosed with GDM (Mauricio et al 1996). As a high-risk group for type 1 diabetes, women with previous autoimmune GDM may be candidates for potential immune intervention strategies (Mauricio et al 2001).

4.3. Cellular immune response and gestational diabetes

There is a significant increase in the absolute number of total and activated (CD3+HLA-DR+) T lymphocytes and a significant increase in the absolute number and percentage of suppressor/cytotoxic T lymphocytes (CD8) and NK lymphocytes (CD57) in GDM patients compared with normal pregnant controls (Mahmoud et al.2006). Concerning frequency for HLA A, B, C, DR antigens in the GDM population, only Cw_7 was found to be significantly increased and A_{10} significantly decreased in comparison with controls (Lapolla et al 1996). When compared with healthy pregnant women, both GDM cohorts showed higher percentages CD4+CD25+ ($P < 0.05$), CD4+CD45RO+ ($P < 0.05$) and CD4+CD29+ (Mahmoud et al 2005).

http://dx.doi.org/10.5772/55634

5. The placenta is a target of cytokines: maternal and fetal influences

There is a robust cytokine network in the placenta with diverse pathogenesis and effects on the development of the fetus.

5.1. Bidirectional nature of cytokine at the fetal-maternal interface

Subpopulations of T helper lymphocytes (CD3+/CD4+) can be classified as either T helper 1 (Th1) or T helper 2 (Th2) cells depending on their cytokine profiles. Th2 cells selectively produce interleukins (IL)-4, IL-5, IL-6, IL-9, IL-10 and IL-13, and are involved in the development of humoral immunity against extracellular pathogens but inhibit several functions of phagocytic cells. In contrast to this, Th1 cells produce interferon-γ (IFN-γ), IL-2 and tumour necrosis factor-α (TNF-α) and evoke cell-mediated immunity and phagocyte-dependent inflammation (Mosmann et al 1989, Mosmann and Moore 1991, Romagnani 2000). Cytokines are mainly produced by cells of the immune system, NK cells, and macrophages in response to an external stimulus such as stress, injury, and infection. Adipose tissue represents an additional source of cytokines, making possible a functional cooperation between the immune system and metabolism (Guerre-Miller 2004, Radaelli et al. 2005).

5.2. The role of adipokines and other inflammatory markers

Research has recently focused on a group of substances produced mainly by adipose tissue called adipokines, this group includes, among others, adiponectin, leptin, Retinol-Binding Protein-4 (RBP-4), and resistin. These substances as well as other inflammatory mediators (CRP, IL-6, PAI-1, TNF-α) seem to play an important role in glucose tolerance and insulin sensitivity dysregulation in women with GDM (Thyfault et al 2005, Defalu 2009). There are two main pathways leading to GDM and T2DM: insulin resistance and chronic subclinical inflammation. Insulin resistance is caused by the inability of tissues to respond to insulin and the deficient secretion of insulin by pancreatic beta cells (Vrachnis et al 2012). Inflammatory processes have a robust contribution to the pathogenesis of dysglycemia condition and acute phase inflammatory response is a risk factor for T2DM and cardiovascular disease [Pickup et al. 2004]. Obesity has a role in the development of both T2DM and GDM through chronic subclinical inflammation, low-grade activation of the acute phase response, and dysregulation of adipokines (Yudkin et al 1999, Greenberg et al 2002). Increased levels of inflammatory agents during and after pregnancy have been reported in patients with GDM, while increased body fat has been strongly associated with inflammation and adipocyte necrosis, hypoxia, and release of chemokines which cause macrophages to infiltrate adipose tissue. Macrophages secrete cytokines which activate the subsequent secretion of inflammation mediating agents, specifically interleukin-6 (IL-6) and C-reactive protein (CRP) (Festa et al 2000). Other molecules such as Plasminogen Activator Inhibitor 1 (PAI-1) and sialic acid lead to dysregulations of metabolism, hyperglycemia, insulin resistance, and diabetes. These are a group of substances that are produced mainly in the adipose tissue. The group includes leptin, adiponectin, tumor necrosis factor alpha (TNF-α), retinol-binding protein-4 (RBP-4), resistin, visfatin, and apelin. These molecules are involved in a wide range of physiological processes including lipid metabolism, atherosclerosis, blood pressure regulation, insulin sensitivity, and angiogenesis, while they also influence immunity and inflammation. Their levels in pathologic states appear increased, with the exception of adiponectin which shows decreased levels (Vrachnis et al 2012).

5.3. Adiponectin

Since the discovery of adiponectin in 1994 by Jeffrey M. Friedman (Zhang et al 1994), more than 20 members of the adiponectin family have been identified (Klein et al 2002, Housa et al 2006). Adiponectin is a 30-kDa protein that is synthesized almost exclusively by adipocytes. It exists in three major oligomeric forms: a low-molecular-weight trimer, a middle-molecular-weight hexamer and high-molecular-weight (HMW) 12- to 18-mer adiponectin. It is an insulin-sensitizing and stimulates glucose uptake in skeletal muscle and reduces hepatic glucose production through AMP-activated protein kinase[Zavalza et al 2008]. Circulating adiponectin levels are reduced in patients with GDM as compared to healthy pregnant controls. Adiponectin mRNA is downregulated in placental tissue, while circulating adiponectin concentrations are decreased postpartum in women with a history of GDM. It also possesses antiatherogenic and anti-inflammatory properties [Chandran et al 2003, Wiecek et al 2007]. The levels of adiponectin decrease as visceral fat increases [Cnop etal 2003, Weyer et al 2001, Hotta et al 2000, Shondorf et. al 2005] in such conditions as central obesity, insulin resistance, and diabetes mellitus. Reduced adiponectin levels have notably been associated with subclinical inflammation [Retnakaran et al 2003]. It has been shown that adiponectin levels begin to decrease early in the pathogenesis of diabetes, as adipose tissue increases in tandem with reduction in insulin sensitivity [Hotta et al 2001]. Hypoadiponectinemia has also been associated with beta cell dysfunction [Musso et al 2005, Retnakaran et al 2005)], while it has additionally been linked to future development of insulin resistance and type 2 diabetes mellitus, in the development of which adiponectin appears to have a causative role (Stefan et al 2002). As such, adiponectin may play a key role in mediating insulin resistance and beta cell dysfunction in the pathogenesis of diabetes (Retnakaran et al 2004, Retnakaran et al 2005). Retnakaran and Associates (2005) have demonstrated that adiponectin concentration is an independent correlate of pancreatic beta cell function in late pregnancy.

5.4. Leptin

Leptin is a 16-kDa protein hormone that is known to play a key role in the regulation of energy intake and energy expenditure and in a number of physiological processes including regulation of endocrine function, inflammation, immune response, reproduction and angiogenesis. The main function of leptin in the human body is the regulation of energy expenditure and control of appetite. Indeed, lack of leptin in mice with a mutation in the gene encoding leptin, or absence of functional leptin receptor (*db*/*db* mice) results in obesity and many associated metabolic complications such as insulin resistance [Ceddia et al 2002)]. Leptin is a key molecule in obesity and it is predominantly produced by white adipose tissue [Harvey and Ashford 2003]. Circulating leptin is actively transported through the blood-brain barrier and acts on the hypothalamic satiety center to decrease food intake. Serum level of leptin reflects the amount of energy stored in the adipose tissue and proportional to body fat mass [Fruhbeck 2006], i.e. increased in obese and decreased after several months of pronounced weight loss [Moschen et al 2009, Hegyi et al 2004]. Thus, it increases insulin sensitivity by influencing insulin secretion, glucose utilization, glycogen synthesis and fatty acid metabolism, regulates gonadotrophin releasing hormone secretion from the hypothalamus and activates the sympathetic nervous system. Leptin acts via transmembrane receptors (OB-R), which belong to the class I cytokine receptor family, such as the receptors of interleukin-2 (IL-2), IL-3, IL-4, IL-6, IL-11, IL-12, granulocyte colony-stimulating factor (G-CSF) or leukemia inhibitory factor (LIF). OB-Rb has full signaling capabilities and is able to activate the JAK/STAT pathway, the major pathway used by leptin to exert its effects [Cirillo et al 2008]. It has receptors on many other cell types such as adipocytes, osteoclasts, endothelial cells, lung and kidney cells, mononuclear blood cells, muscle, endometrial and liver cells [Hegyi et al 2004].

5.5. Association between leptin and TNF-alpha and insulin resistance

Placental leptin mRNA production is upregulated by tumour necrosis factor (TNF) α and interleukin (IL)-6. Most studies have found increased leptin concentrations in GDM. Moreover, hyperleptinaemia in early pregnancy appears to be predictive of an increased risk to develop GDM later in pregnancy independent of maternal adiposity (Hotamistigil et al 1993, Das 2002, Kirwan et al 2002,). The human placenta expresses virtually all known cytokines including tumor necrosis factor (TNF)-α, resistin, and leptin, which are also produced by the adipose cells (Qasim etal 2008, Rabe et al. 2008). The discovery that some of these adipokines as key players in the regulation of insulin action suggests possible novel interactions between the placenta and adipose tissue in understanding pregnancy-induced insulin resistance, which is evident in gestational diabetes mellitus (GDM) (Winzer et al 2004).

5.6. Inflammatory mediators in diabetes mellitus

Gestational diabetes mellitus is characterized by an amplification of the low-grade inflammation already existing in normal pregnancy (Retnakaran et al 2010). This hypothesis is supported by increased circulating concentrations of inflammatory molecules like TNFα and IL-6 in GDM pregnancies. TNFα is one of the candidate molecules responsible for causing insulin resistance. Comparison of the placental gene expression profile between normal and diabetic pregnancies indicates that increased leptin synthesis in GDM is associated with a higher production of proinflammatory cytokines, e.g. IL-6 and TNFα causing a chronic inflammatory environment that enhances leptin production (Pickup et al 2000, Winkler et al 2002, Gao et al 2008). Thus, compared with normal pregnant women, placental leptin expression in patients with GDM is increased. Conversely, leptin itself increases production of TNFα and IL-6 by monocytes and stimulates the production of CC-chemokine ligands. Elevated leptin concentrations in turn amplify inflammation

6. Link between inflammation and insulin resistance

In 1876 Ebstein asserted that sodium salicylate could make the symptoms of diabetes mellitus totally disappear. Similarly, in 1901 Williamson found that "sodium salicylate had a definite influence in greatly diminishing the sugar excretion"(Shoelson 2002, Shoelson et al 2006, Cefalu 2009). Increased levels of markers and mediators of inflammation and acute-phase reactants such as fibrinogen, C-reactive protein (CRP), IL-6, plasminogen activator inhibitor-1 (PAI-1), sialic acid, and white cell count correlate with incident T2D (Sternberg et al 1992, Bo et al 2005, Kim et al. 2008). Markers of inflammation and coagulation are reduced with intensive lifestyle intervention. This was confirmed in the diabetes prevention program (DPP Research Group 2005). Experimental evidence have also confirmed that adipose tissue–derived proinflammatory cytokines such as TNF-α could actually cause insulin resistance (Wolf et al 2003, Dandona et al 2004, Hu et al 2004, Heitritter et al 2005). Hotamisligil and colleagues (1993, 1994) and Karasik and Colleagues (1993) first showed that the proinflammatory cytokine TNF-α was able to induce insulin resistance. The concept of fat as a site for the production of cytokines and other bioactive substances quickly extended beyond TNF-α to include leptin, IL-6, resistin, monocyte chemoattractant protein-1 (MCP-1), PAI-1, angiotensinogen, visfatin, retinol-binding protein-4, serum amyloid A (SAA), and others (Dandona et al 2004). Adiponectin is similarly produced by fat, but expression decreases with increased adiposity. While leptin and adiponectin are true adipokines that appear to be produced exclusively by adipocytes, TNF-α, IL-6, MCP-1, visfatin, and PAI-1 are expressed as well at high levels in activated macrophages and/or other cells(Baer et al 1998). Sites of resistin production are more complex; they include macrophages in humans but both adipocytes and macrophages in rodents. TNF-α, IL-6, resistin, and other pro- or antiinflammatory cytokines appear to participate in the induction and maintenance of the subacute inflammatory state associated with obesity (Thyfault et al 2005). MCP-1 and other chemokines have essential roles in the recruitment of macrophages to adipose tissue. These cytokines and chemokines activate intracellular pathways that promote the development of insulin resistance and T2D (Wu et al 2002, de Victoria et al. 2009).

6.1. Mechanisms of insulin resistance by pro-inflammatory cytokines

The JNK (also referred to as SAPK) and p38 MAPKs are members of the complex superfamily of MAP serine/threonine protein kinases. This superfamily also includes the ERKs (Lewis et al 1998). In contrast to ERKs (also referred to as MAPKs), which are typically activated by mitogens, JNK/SAPK and p38 MAPK are known as stress-activated kinases. This can be attributed to the fact that the activities of these enzymes are stimulated by a variety of exogenous and endogenous stress-inducing stimuli including hyperglycemia, ROS, oxidative stress, osmotic stress, proinflammatory cytokines, heat shock, and UV irradiation (Tibbles et al 1999). Many of the more typical proinflammatory stimuli simultaneously activate JNK and

IKKβ pathways, including cytokines and TLRs (Seger and Krebs 1995). Concordantly, genetic or chemical inhibition of either JNK or IKKβ/NF-κB can improve insulin resistance. The several mechanisms have been postulated to explain how obesity activates JNK and NF-κB. These can be separated into receptor (Lowes et al 2002) and nonreceptor pathways (Tamura et al 2002). Proinflammatory cytokines such as TNF-α and IL-1β activate JNK and IKKβ/NF-κB through classical receptor-mediated mechanisms that have been well characterized (Shen et al 2001, Tournier et al 2001). JNK and IKKβ/NF-κB are also activated by pattern recognition receptors, defined as surface proteins that recognize foreign substances. These include the Toll-like receptors (TLRs) and the receptor for advanced glycation end products (RAGE). Many TLR ligands are microbial products, including LPS and lipopeptides (Tamura et al 2002).

6.2. Transcription versus phosphorylation in the pathogenesis of insulin resistance

JNK is a stress kinase that normally phosphorylates the c-Jun component of the AP-1 transcription factor, but to date there are no known links between this well-established transcriptional pathway and JNK-induced insulin resistance. JNK has been shown to promote insulin resistance through the phosphorylation of serine residues (Shen et al 2001, Tournier et al 2001). Insulin receptor signaling that normally occurs through a tyrosine kinase cascade is inhibited by counterregulatory serine/threonine phosphorylations.

6.3. IKK β signaling pathway and insulin resistance

Unlike JNK, IKKβ does not phosphorylate IRS-1 to cause insulin resistance but causes insulin resistance through transcriptional activation of NF-κB. Increased lipid deposition in adipocytes leads to the production of proinflammatory cytokines, including TNF-α, IL-6, IL-1β, and resistin, which further activate JNK and NF-κB pathways through a feed-forward mechanism (Hou et al 2008). In addition to the cytokines, there is upregulated expression of transcriptions factors, receptors, and other relevant proteins including chemokines that recruit monocytes and stimulate their differentiation into macrophages.

Cytokines and chemokines produced locally include MCP-1 and macrophage inflammatory protein-1α (MIP-1α), MIP-1β, MIP-2, and MIP-3α. T cell activation leads to expression of IFN-γ and lymphotoxin; macrophages, endothelial cells, and SMCs produce TNF-α; and together these stimulate the local production of IL-6 in the atheroma

6.4. Oxidative stress and activation of JNK and NF-κB pathways

In addition to proinflammatory cytokine and pattern recognition receptors, cellular stresses activate JNK and NF-κB, including ROS and ER stress. Elevated glucose cause oxidative stress through (1) increased production of mitochondrial reactive oxygen species (ROS), (2) Non-enzymatic glycation of proteins, (3) Glucose autoxidation (Elevated free fatty acids (FFA) and beta oxidation (Tibbles et al 1999, Evans et al 2002, Lewis et al 2002. Muoio et al. 2008). Systemic markers of oxidative stress increase with adiposity, consistent with a role for ROS in the development of obesity-induced insulin resistance, (Ozdemir et al 2005). One potential mechanism is through the activation of NADPH oxidase by lipid accumulation in the adipocyte, which increases ROS production. This mechanism was shown to increase the production of TNF-α, IL-6, and MCP-1, and decrease the production of adiponectin (Barbour et al 2007). Consistent with this, the antioxidant *N*-acetyl cysteine can reduce ROS and improve insulin resistance in a hyperglycemia-induced model (Pieper et al 1997, Ozkilic et al 2006). Lipid accumulation also activates the unfolded protein response to increase ER stress in fat and liver. ER stress has been shown to activate JNK and subsequently, lead to serine phosphorylation of insulin receptor substrate-1 (IRS-1), but as with all of the stimuli, ER stress similarly activates NF-$\kappa\beta$ (Evans et al 2002)

7. Health implications of cytokines, lipid metabolism, inflammation and GDM

The triad of cytokines, lipid metabolism and inflammation are hooked together by a biological thread of oxidative stress and pathogenetic end-point of insulin resistance. Oxidative stress inhibits expression of Pax 3, a gene that is essential for neural tube closure, and possibly congenital cardiac anomalies which have been associated with uncontrollable diabetes in pregnancy before and in early pregnancy (Chang et al 2003). The association between GDM and macrosomia is real, with a secondary effect of increased cesarean section and increased risk of postpartum genital infection and development of overt type 2 diabetes mellitus. The markers of inflammation, dyslipidemia, oxidative stress and endothelial dysfunction may provide additional information about a patient's risk of developing cardiovascular disease and hypertension. This may provide new attractive targets for drug development.

8. Intervention strategies

GDM offers an important opportunity for the development for testing and the implementation of clinical strategies in diabetic prevention (Volpe et al 2007). The main objective should be to improve insulin sensitivity and prevent diabetes mellitus.

8.1. Lifestyle modification

Lifestyle modifications have been shown to be successful in decreasing the progression to T2DM in several populations, including American, Finnish and Asian, so it seems rational to consider similar interventions in women with a history of GDM (An Empowered Based Diabetic Prevention 2011). The ACOG (2003), RCOG Guidelines (2011), NICE Guidelines (2009) and the ADA (2005) all recommend that women at increased risk for T2DM should be counseled about the benefits of diet, exercise, and weight reduction and/or maintenance in an effort to prevent the development of T2DM as part of preconception care.

8.2. Breast-feeding

Breast-feeding is associated with reduced blood glucose levels and a reduced incidence of T2DM among both women with a history of GDM and women in the general population. Lactation has also been associated with postpartum weight loss, reduced long-term obesity risk, and a lower prevalence of the metabolic syndrome (O'Reilly et al 2003).

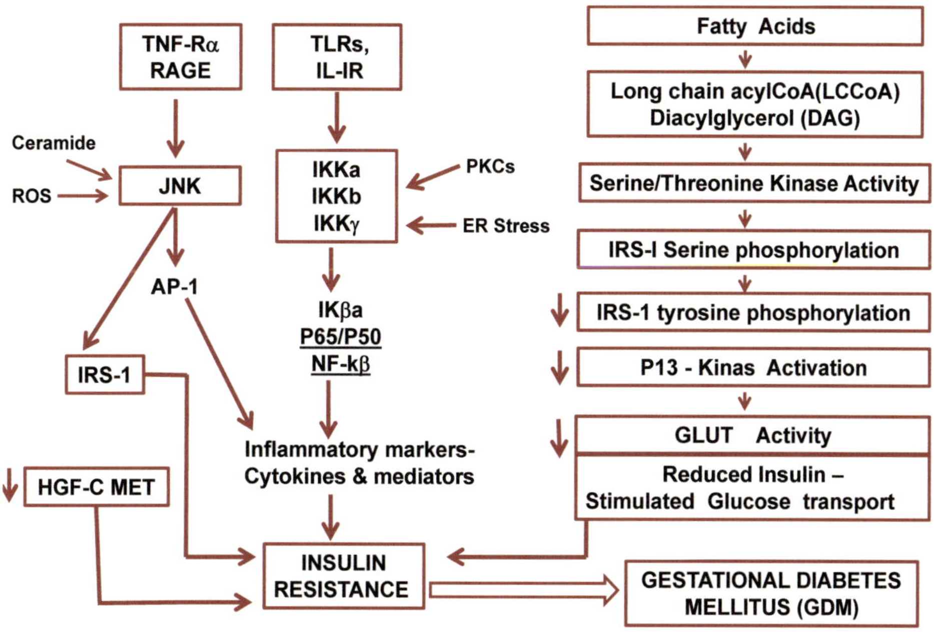

References: Shoelson et al 2006, Qatanani et al 2007, Savage et al 2007)

Figure 1. Mechanisms of Insulin Resistance and Gestational diabetes Fatty acid metabolites (long-chain acyl-CoA [LCCoA] and diacylglycerol [DAG]) trigger a serine/threonine kinase cascade andl protein kinase C, to induce serine/threonine phosphorylation. This inhibits IRS-1 binding and activation of PI 3-kinase and insulin signalling with resultant reduced insulin-stimulated glucose transport. Obesity-associated changes in secretion of adipokines and inflammatory IKKβ and NF-kβ and JNK pathways through ligands for TNF-α, IL-1, Toll and AGE receptors, intracellular stresses like Reactive oxygen species,Ceramide and PKC isoforms. These factors modulate insulin signalling, through activation of NF-kβ and cause insulin Resistance(Shoelson et al 2006, Qatanani et al 2007, Savage et al 2007,)

8.3. Pharmacologic interventions

Insulin is the drug to use, especially in GDM. Drugs with anti-inflammatory and vascular effects have future potential of being used in interventions aimed at reducing the enormous cardiovascular burden associated with Type 2 diabetes (Ziegler 2005). Use of sodium salicylate (Aspirin) (Hostamistigil et al 1993, Karasik et al 1993) has the concerns with high dose and possible side-effect of peptic ulceration. The use of antioxidant E and C reduces embryopathy in animal model (Cederberg) and in human with use of N-acetyl Cysteine has beneficial effects (Ozkilic et al 2006).

9. Concluding remarks

Recent advances in the understanding of carbohydrate metabolism during pregnancy, suggest that preventive measures should be aimed at improving insulin sensitivity in women with strong risk factors of developing GDM. The mechanisms involved in the pathogenesis of insulin resistance and Gestational Diabetes Mellitus are summarized in Figure 1. Further research is needed to elucidate the mechanisms and consequences of alterations in lipid metabolism during pregnancy (Marseille-Tremblay et al 2008). Inflammation-induced insulin resistance is certainly increasing in parallel with the epidemic of obesity. Strategies for reducing this trend should be part of the Public Health initiatives.

9.1. Future directions

There is need for genetic studies especially from the Human Genome to identify those with candidate genes for diabetes and epigenetic factors that may affect gene expression and predisposition to inflammation. It should be possible to directly target inflammation with pharmacological interventions to treat and/or prevent insulin resistance and T2D and modulate risk for CVD and other metabolic conditions. In addition to anti-inflammatory drugs such as NF-κβ inhibitors and IL-1 receptor antagonists already known to improve inflammatory and glycemic parameters, should have utility to block the prolonged exposure to inflammatory danger signals may further enhance the metabolic and cardiovascular outcome of obese patients. Early recognition and management of women predisposed to develop T2DM is crucial in the development of primary health care strategies, modification of lifestyle, and dietary habits significantly to prevent or delay of insulin resistance and development of glucose intolerance.

Author details

Alexander E. Omu

Professor of Obstetrics and Gynaecology, and Andrology, Faculty of Medicine, Health Sciences Center, Kuwait University, Kuwait

References

[1] ACOG (2011)-Screening and Diagnosis of Gestational Diabetes Mellitus. No 504.

[2] Ahima S, Flier (S2000). Adipose Tissue as an Endocrine Organ. Trends in Endocrinology & Metabolism 11: 327-332.

[3] Ali S, Dornhorst A (2011). Diabetes in pregnancy: health risks and management. Postgrad Med J 87:417-427

[4] American Diabetes Association (2005). Standards of medical care in diabetes. (Position Statement). Diabetes Care 28 (Suppl) : S4 –S36,

[5] An Empowerment-Based Diabetes Self-management Education Program for Hispanic/Latinos (2011): A Quasi-experimental Pilot Study The Diabetes Educator 37: 770-779

[6] Anger GJ, Piquette-Miller M (2010). Impact of Hyperlipidemia on Plasma Protein Binding and Hepatic Drug Transporter and Metabolic Enzyme Regulation in a Rat Model of Gestational Diabetes. J Pharmacol 334: 21-32 B

[7] Arends NJT, Boostra VH, Duivenvoorden HJ, Hofman PL, Cutfield WS, Hokken-Koelega ACS 2005 Reduced insulin sensitivity and the presence of cardiovascular risk factors in short prepubertal children born small for gestational age (SGA). Clin Endocrinol (Oxf) 62:44–45

[8] Barbour L A, Mccurdy C E, Hernandez T L, Kirwan J P, Catalano P M, Friedman J E (2007). Cellular mechanisms for Insulin Resistance in Normal Pregnancy and Gestational Diabetes Diabetes Care 30: S112-S119

[9] Barker DJ, Martyn CN, Osmond C, Hales CN, Fall CH (1993) Growth in utero and serum cholesterol concentration in adult life. BMJ 307:1524–1527

[10] Behan KJ (2011). New ADA Guidelines for Diagnosis, Screening of Diabetes. Advance Admin. Lab 20:22.

[11] Ben-Haroush A, Yogev Y., Hod M (2004). Epidemiology of gestational diabetes mellitus and its association with Type 2 diabetes. Diabetic Medicine 21: 103–113

[12] Boney CM, Verma A, Tucker R, Vohr BR (2005). Metabolic Syndrome in Childhood: Association With Birth Weight, Maternal Obesity, and Gestational Diabetes Mellitus. 115: e293-e296.

[13] Bray GA, Jablonski KA, Fujimoto WY, Barrett-Connor E, Haffner S, Hanson RL, Hill JO, Hubbard V, Kriska A, Stamm E, Pi-Sunyer FK (2008). Relation of central adiposity and body mass index to the development of diabetes in the Diabetes Prevention Program. Am J Clin Nutr 87:1212–8.

[14] Buchanan TA, Xiang A,. Kjos SL, Watanabe R (2007). What Is Gestational Diabetes? Diabetes Care 30: S105-S111

[15] Butte NF (2000). Carbohydrate and lipid metabolism in pregnancy: normal compared with gestational diabetes mellitus. Am J Clin Nutr. 71(Suppl):1256S-61S.

[16] Canadian Diabetes Association (2003) Clinical practice guidelines for the prevention and management of diabetes in Canada. Can J Diabetes. 27 (suppl 2):S151-S156.

[17] Casanueva E, Viteri FE (2003). Iron and oxidative stress in pregnancy. Journal of Nutrition 133:1700S–1708S.

[18] Catalano PM, Nizielski S, Shao J, Preston L, Qiao L, Friedman JE (2002). Down-regulated IRS-1 and PPARgamma in obese women with gestational diabetes: relationship to FFA during pregnancy. Am J Physiol Endocrinol Metab 282:E522–E533.

[19] Chandran M, Phillips SA, Ciaraldi T, Henry RR. Adiponectin: more than just another fat cell hormone? Diabetes Care. 2003;26(8):2442–2450.

[20] Cederberg J, Siman CM, Eriksson UJ (2001). Combined treatment with vitamins E and C decrease oxidative stress and improves fetal outcome in experimental diabetic pregnancy. Pediatric Research 49: 755–762.

[21] Cefalu WT (2009). Inflammation, Insulin Resistance and Type 2 Diabetes: Back to the future. Diabetes 58:307-308

[22] Chang T.I, Horal M, Jain SK, Wang F, Patel R, Loeken MR (2003). Oxidant regulation of gene expression and neural tube development: Insights gained from diabetic pregnancy on molecular causes of neural of neural tube defects. Diabetologia 46:538-545.

[23] Cigolini M, Tonoli M, Borgato L, Frigotto L, Manzato F, Zeminian S, Cardinale C, Camin M, Chiaramonte E, DeSandre G, and Lunardi C (1999). Expression of plasminogen activator inhibitor-1 in human adipose tissue: a role for TNF-α? Atherosclerosis 143: 81–90,

[24] Cnop M, Havel PJ, Utzschneider KM, Carr DB, Sinha MK, Boyko EJ, Retzlaff BM, Knopp RH, Brunzell JD, Kahn SE (2003). Relationship of adiponectin to body fat distribution, insulin sensitivity and plasma lipoproteins: evidence for independent roles of age and sex. Diabetologia. 46:459–469.

[25] Coppack SW (2001). Pro-inflammatory cytokines and adipose tissue. Proc Nutr Soc 60: 349–356,

[26] Coughlin MT, Vervaart PP, Permezel M, Georgiou HM, Rice GE (2004). Altered placental oxidative stress gestational diabetes mellitus. Placenta 25:78–84.

[27] Damn P. (1998). Gestational diabetes mellitus and subsequent development of overt diabetes mellitus. Danish Medical Bulletin 45:495–509

[28] Darmady J, Postle A. Lipid metabolism in pregnancy. BJOG 1982; 89:211-215.

[29] de Leiva A, Mauricio D and Corcoy R. Immunology of gestational diabetes mellitus. 2008, Pages 100-106. In Textbook of Diabetes and Pregnancy, Edited Moshe Hod MD, Lois Jovanovic, Gian Carlo Di Renzo, Alberto de Leiva, and. Second Edition.

[30] Davi G, Patrono C (2005). Lipid peroxidation in Diabetes. Antioxid Redox Signal 7:256-266.

[31] De Victoria E O M, Xu X, Koska J, Francisco AM, Scalise M, Ferrante AW Jr, Krakoff J (2009). Macrophage Content in Subcutaneous Adipose Tissue Associations With

http://dx.doi.org/10.5772/55634

Adiposity, Age, Inflammatory Markers, and Whole-Body Insulin Action in Healthy Pima Indians. Diabetes 58:385-393.

[32] Demirci C, Ernst S, Alvarez-Perez J C., Rosa T, Valle S, Shridhar V, Casinelli G P. Alonso L C., Vasavada R C., and García-Ocana A (2012). Loss of HGF/c-Met Signaling in Pancreatic β-Cells Leads to Incomplete Maternal β-Cell Adaptation and Gestational Diabetes Mellitus Diabetes 61:1143-1152

[33] Dooley SL, Metzger BE, Cho NH (1991). Gestational diabetes mellitus: influence of race on disease prevalence and perinatal outcome in a U.S. population. Diabetes 40: S25–S29.

[34] El-Assaad W, Buteau J, Peyot MC, Nolan C, Roduit R, Hardy S, Joly E, Dhaibo G, Rosenberg L, Prentki M (2003). Saturated fatty acids synergise with elevated glucose to cause pancreatic beta cell death. Endocrinology 144: 4154-4163

[35] Eriksson K and Lindgärde F (1991). Prevention of Type 2 (non-insulin-dependent) diabetes mellitus by diet and physical exercise The 6-year Malmö feasibility study Diabetologia 34:891-898.

[36] Ernst S, Demirci C, Valle S, Velazquez-Garcia S, Garcia-Ocada A (2011). Mechanisms of adaptation of maternal beta cells during pregnancy. Diabetic Manag 1: 239-248

[37] Evans JL, Goldfine ID, Maddux BA and Grodsky GM (2002). Oxidative Stress and Stress-Activated Signaling Pathways: A Unifying Hypothesis of Type 2 Diabetes. Endocrine Reviews 23: 599-622.

[38] Ferber KM, Keller E, Albert ED, Ziegler AG (1999). Predictive Value of Human Leukocyte Antigen Class II Typing for the Development of Islet Autoantibodies and Insulin-Dependent Diabetes Postpartum in Women with Gestational Diabetes. J. Clin Endocrinol & Metab 84: 2342-2348

[39] Festa A, Agostino R. D Jr, Howard G, Mykkänen L, Tracy R. P., and Haffner S. M. (2000). Chronic subclinical inflammation as part of the insulin resistance syndrome: the insulin resistance atherosclerosis study (IRAS). Circulation 102: 42–47.

[40] Freinkel N, Metzger BE, Phelps RL, Simpson JL, Martin AO, Radvany R, Ober C, Dooley SL, Depp RO, Belton A (1986). Gestational diabetes mellitus: a syndrome with phenotypic and genotypic heterogeneity. Horm Metab Res 18:427–430.

[41] Gallagher D, Kelley DE, Yim J E, Spence N, Albu J, Boxt L, Pi-Sunyer F X and Heshka S (2009). Adipose tissue distribution is different in type 2 diabetes. Am J Clin Nutr. 89: 807–814.

[42] Gao XL, Yang HX, Zhao Y (2008). Variations of tumor necrosis factor-α, leptin and adiponectin in mid-trimester of gestational diabetes mellitus. Chinese Medical Journal. 121: 701–705.

[43] Qatanani M, Lazar MA (2007). Mechanisms of obesity-associated insulin resistance: many choices on the menu. Genes & Dev 21: 1443-1445

[44] Gonzalez-Clemente J.M, Carro O, Gallach I, Vioque J, Humanes A, Suaret C, Abella M, Gimenez-Perez G, Mauricio D (2007). Increased cholesterol intake in women with gestational diabetes mellitus. Diabetes & Metabolism 33: 25-29.

[45] Greenberg A. S and McDaniel M L(2002). Identifying the links between obesity, insulin resistance and β-cell function: potential role of adipocyte-derived cytokines in the pathogenesis of type 2 diabetes. Euro J Clin Invest 32, supplement 3: 24–34.

[46] Guerre-Miller M (2004). Adipose tissue and adipokines: for better or worse. Diabete Metab 30:13–19.

[47] Hanachi P, Moghadam RH, Latiffah AL(2009). Investigation of Lipid Profiles and Lipid Peroxidation in Patients with Type 2 Diabetes. European Journal of Scientific Research 28; 6-13

[48] Hanna FWF, Peters JR, Harlow J and Jones PW (2008). Gestational diabetes screening and glycaemic management; Q J. Med 101: 777-784.

[49] Harvey J, Ashford ML (2003). Leptin in the CNS: much more than a satiety signal. Neuropharmacology 44: 845–854.

[50] Hedley A A, Ogden C L, Johnson C L, Carroll M.D, Curtin L R (2004). Overweight and Obesity Among U.S. Children, Adolescents and Adults, 1999-2002. J. Am. Med Ass. 291: 2847-2850.

[51] Heinig J, Wilhelm S, Müller H, Briese V, Bittorf T, Brock J (2000). Determination of cytokine mRNA-expression in term human placenta of patients with gestational hypertension, intrauterine growth retardation and gestational diabetes mellitus using polymerase chain reaction. Zentralbl Gynakol. 122: 413-8.

[52] Hostamistigil GS, Shargill NS, Spiegelman BM (1994). Adipose expression of tumour necrosis factor alpha BM.Altered gene expression for tumour necrosis factor alpha and its receptors during drug and dietary modulation of insulin resistance. Endocrinology 134;264-270

[53] Hotamisligil GS, Spiegelman BM (1994). Tumor necrosis factor α: a key component of the obesity-diabetes link. Diabetes. 43:1271–1278.

[54] Hotta K, Funahashi T, Arita Y, Takahashi M, Matsuda M, Okamoto Y, Iwahashi H, Kuriyama H, Ouchi N, Maeda K, Nishida M, Kihara S, Sakai N, Nakajima T, Hasegawa K, Muraguchi M, Ohmoto Y, Nakamura T, Yamashita S, Hanafusa T, Matsuzawa Y (2000). Plasma concentrations of a novel, adipose-specific protein, adiponectin, in type 2 diabetic patients. Arteriosclerosis, Thrombosis, and Vascular Biology. 20: 1595–1599.

[55] Hotta K, Funahashi T, Bodkin NL, Ortmeyer HK, Arita Y, Hansen BC, Matsuzawa Y (2001). Circulating concentrations of the adipocyte protein adiponectin are decreased

in parallel with reduced insulin sensitivity during the progression to type 2 diabetes in rhesus monkeys. Diabetes 50: 1126–1133.

[56] Hou Y, Karin FL and Ostrowski MC (2008). Analysis of the IKKβ/NF-κB Signaling Pathway during Embryonic Angiogenesis. Dev Dyn. 237: 2926–2935.

[57] Housa D, Housova J, Vernerova Z, Haluzik M (2006). Adipocytokines and cancer. Physiol Res 55:233-244.

[58] Hunt JS, Petroff MG, McIntire RH, Ober C (2005). HLA-G and immune tolerance in pregnancy. The FASEB J. 19: 681-693

[59] Hutley L, Prins J (2005). Fat as an endocrine organ: Relationship to the Metabolic Syndrome Am. J Med Sc 330: 280-289.

[60] Hyperglycemia and Adverse Pregnancy Outcome (HAPO) Study (2009. Associations with neonatal anthropometrics. Diabetes 58:453–459

[61] Jensen MD (2006). Adipose tissue as an endocrine: implication of its distribution on free fatty acid metabolism. Eur. Heart J. Supplement B: S813-S819.

[62] Karazik A, Rothenberg PL, Yamada K, White MF, Khan CR. J (1990).The proinflammatory cytokines with inflammation expression: TNF-alpha, IL-6 and MCP-1 in Macrophages. Biol Chem 265: 10225-10231.

[63] Kautzky-Willer A, Krssk M, Winzer C, Pacini G, Tura A, Farhan S et al (2003). Increased intramyocellular lipid concentrationidentifies impaired glucose metabolism in women with previous gestational diabetes. Diabetes 52: 244-251.

[64] Kershaw EE, Flier JS (2004). Adipose tissue as an endocrine organ. J Clin Endocrinol Metab 89: 2548-2556.

[65] Kirwan JP, Hauguel-de Mouzon S, Lepercy J, Kallan SC, Catalano PM (2002). TNF-alpha is a predictor of insulin resistance in human pregnancy. Diabetes 51: 2207-2213.

[66] Kjos SL, Buchanan TA (1999). Gestational diabetes mellitus. N. Engl. J. Med. 341:1749–1756.

[67] Klein C J, Dyck P J B, Friedenberg S M, Burns T M, Windebank A J, Dyck P J (2002), Inflammation and neuropathic attacks in hereditary brachial plexus neuropathyJ Neurol Neurosurg Psychiatry 73:45-50

[68] Koukkou E, Watts G, Lowy C (1996). Serum lipid, lipoprotein and apolipoprotein changes in gestational diabetes mellitus: a cross-sectional and prospective study. J Clin Pathol 49:634–637,

[69] Lambrinoudaki I, Vlachou SA, Creatsas G (2010). Genetics in gestational diabetes mellitus: association with incidence, severity, pregnancy outcome and response to treatment. Curr Diabetes Rev. 6: 393-399.

[70] Lauenborg J, Hansen T, Jansen DM, Vestergaard H, Molstad-PedersenI, Hornnes P, Locht H, Pedersen O, Damm P (2004). Increasing incidence of of diabetes after gesta-

tional diabetes: a long-term follow-up in a Dannish population. Diabetes Care 27: 1194-1199

[71] Lapolla A, Betterle C., Sanzari M., Zanchetta R., Pfeifer E., Businaro A., et al (1996). An immunological and genetic study of patients with gestational diabetes mellitus Acta Diabetologica 33: 139-144.

[72] Lapolla A, Dalfrà MG, Fedele D (2009). Diabetes related autoimmunity in gestational diabetes mellitus: is it important? Nutr Metab Cardiovasc Dis. 19: 674-82

[73] Lewis G F, Carpentier A, Adeli K and Giacca A (2002). Disordered Fat Storage and Mobilization in the Pathogenesis of Insulin Resistance and Type 2 Diabetes. Endocrine Reviews23: 2 201-229

[74] Lo JC, Feigenbaum SL, Escobar JE,Yang J, Crites Y M, Ferrara A (2006). Increased Prevalence of Gestational Diabetes Mellitus Among Women With Diagnosed Polycystic Ovary Syndrome. A population-based study. Diabetes Care 29: 1915-1919.

[75] Löbner K, Knopff A, Baumgarten A, Mollenhauer U, Marienfeld S, Garrido-Franco M, Bonifacio E, Ziegler AG (2006). Predictors of Postpartum Diabetes in Women With Gestational Diabetes Mellitus. Diabetes 55: 792-797

[76] Love-Gregory L, Permutt MA (2007). HNF4A genetic variants: role in diabetes Curr. Opin Clin Nutr Metab Care. 10: 397-402.

[77] Lowes VL, Ip NY, Wong YH (2002), Integration of signals from receptor tyrosine kinases and G protein-coupled receptors. NeuroSignals 11:5-19.

[78] Mahmoud F, Abul H, Omu A, Haines D (2005). Lymphocyte sub-populations in gestational diabetes. Am J Reprod Immunol. 53: 21-9.

[79] Mahmoud FF, Haines DD, Abul HT, Omu AE, Abu-Donia MB (2006). Butyrylcholinesterase activity in gestational diabetes: correlation with lymphocyte subpopulations in peripheral blood. Am J. Reprod Immunol 56:186–192.

[80] Mauricio D, Balsells M, Morales J, Corcoy R, Puig-Domingo M, de Leiva A (1996). Islet cell autoimmunity in women with gestational diabetes and risk of progression to insulin-dependent diabetes mellitus. Diabetes Metab Rev 12:275–285.

[81] Mauricio D, de Leiva A (2001). Autoimmune gestational diabetes mellitus: a distinct clinical entity? Diabetes Metab Res Rev. 17: 422-428.

[82] Marseille-Tremblay C, Ethier-Chiasson M, Forest J C, Giguère Y, Masse A, Mounier C, Lafond J (2008). Impact of maternal circulating cholesterol and gestational diabetes mellitus on lipid metabolism in human term placenta. Molecular Reproduction and Development 75: 1054–1062.

[83] Merzouk H, Bouchenak M, Loukidi B, Madani S, Prost J, Belleville J (2000). Fetal macrosomia related to maternal poorly controlled type 1 diabetes strongly impairs serum lipoprotein concentrations and composition. J Clin Pathol 53:917–923.

[84] Metzger BE, Gabbe SG, Persson B, Buchanan TA, Catalano PA, Damm P, Dyer AR, Leiva A, Hoc M, Kitzmiller JL, Lowe LP, McIntyre HD, Oats JJ, Omori Y, Schmidt MI(2010). International association of diabetes and pregnancy study groups recommendations on the diagnosis and classification of hyperglycemia in pregnancy. International Association of Diabetes and Pregnancy Study Groups Consensus Panel Diabetes Care 33:676– 682.

[85] Mortaz M, Fewtrell MS, Cole TJ, Lucas A (2001). Birth weight, subsequent growth, and cholesterol metabolism in children 8–12 years old born preterm. Arch Dis Child 84:212–217

[86] Moschen AR, Kaser A, Enrich B, Mosheimer B, Theurl M, Niederegger H, Tilg H (2007). Visfatin, an adipocytokine with proinflammatory and immunomodulating properties. J Immunol. 178:1748-58.

[87] Mosmann, T.R. and Coffman, R.L. (1989) Th1 and Th2 cells; different patterns of lymphokine secretion lead to different functional properties. Annu. Rev. Immunol 7: 145–173.

[88] Mosmann, J. and Moore, K. (1991) The role of IL-10 in crossregulation of TH1 and TH2 response. Immunol. Today 12: A49-A53.

[89] Muoio DM, Newgard GB (2008). Fatty Acid Oxidation and Insulin Action. When Less Is More. Diabetes 57: 1455-1456

[90] Musso G, Gambino R, Biroli G, Carello M, Faga E, Pacini G, De Michieli F, Cassader M, Durazzo M, Rizzetto M, Pagano G (2005). Hypoadiponectinemia predicts the severity of hepatic fibrosis and pancreatic Beta-cell dysfunction in nondiabetic nonobese patients with nonalcoholic steatohepatitis. Am J Gastroenterol. 100:2438–2446.

[91] O'Reilly M W, Avalos G, Dennedy M C and Dunne F (2011). Atlantic DIP: high prevalence of abnormal glucose tolerance postpartum is reduced by breast-feeding in women with prior gestational diabetes mellitus. Eur J Endocrinol.165: 953-959.

[92] O'Sullivan JB (1991). Diabetes Mellitus after GDM. Diabetes 40:131-135.

[93] Omu A E, Al-Azemi M K, Omu F E, Fatinikun T, Abraham S, George S, Mahnazhath N (2010). Butyrylcholinesterase activity in women with diabetes mellitus in pregnancy: Correlation with antioxidant activity. J Obstet Gynaecol. 30: 122-6

[94] Omu AE. Unravelling the Connection Between Gestational Diabetes Mellitus and Butyrylcholinesterase. Chapter 12. In Gestational Diabetes Mellitus, Ed. Miroslav Radenkovic. InTech 2011. Rijeka, Croatia.

[95] Ozdemir G, Ozden M, Maral H, Kuskay S, Cetinalp P, Tarkun I (2005). Malondialdehyde, glutathione, glutathione peroxidase and homocysteine levels in type 2 diabetic patients with and without microalbuminuria. Ann Clin Biochem. 42: 99-104.

[96] Ozkilic AC, Cengiz M, Ozaydin A, Cobanoglu A, Kanigur G (2006). The role of N-acetylcysteine treatment on anti-oxidative status in patients with type II diabetes mellitus. J Basic Clin Physiol Pharmacol 17:245-54.

[97] NICE Clinical Guidelines (2008). Diabetes in Pregnancy. No. 63.

[98] Pickup JC (2004). Inflammation and activated innate immunity in the pathogenesis of type 2 diabetes. Diabetes Care. 27: 813–823.

[99] Pickup JC, Chusney GD, Thomas SM, Burt D (2000). Plasma interleukin-6, tumour necrosis factor α and blood cytokine production in type 2 diabetes. Life Sciences. 67: 291–300.

[100] Pieper GM, Riaz UH (1997);. Activation of nuclear factor-kappaB in cultured endothelial cells by increased glucose concentration: prevention by calphostin. C. J Cardiovasc Pharmacol. 30:528–532.

[101] Radaelli T, Uvena-Celebrezze J, Minium J, Huston-Presley L, Catalano P, Hauguel de Mouzon S (2005). Maternal interleukin-6, a marker of fetal growth and adiposity. J Soc Gynecol Invest 13:53–57.

[102] RCOG (2011). Diagnosis and Treatment of Gestational Diabetes: SAC Opinion Paper 23.

[103] Retnakaran R, Hanley AJ, Raif N, Connelly PW, Sermer M, Zinman B (2003). C-reactive protein and gestational diabetes: the central role of maternal obesity. J. Clin. Endocrinol. Metab. 88:3507–3512.

[104] Retnakaran R, Hanley AJG, Raif N, Connelly PW, Sermer M, Zinman B (2004). Reduced adiponectin concentration in women with gestational diabetes: a potential factor in progression to type 2 diabetes. Diabetes Care 27: 799–800

[105] Retnakaran R, Hanley AJG, Raif N, HimingCR, Connelly PW, Sermer M, Kahn SE, Zimman B (2005). Adiponectin and beta cell dysfunction in gestational diabetes: pathophysiological implications. Diabetologia 48:993–1001

[106] Romagnani S (2000). T-cell subsets (Th1 versus Th2). Ann. Allergy Asthma Immunol 85: 9–18.

[107] Savage DB, Petersen KF, Shulman GI. Disordered lipid metabolism and the pathogenesis of insulin resistance. Physiol Rev. 2007;87:507–520.

[108] Schaefer-Graf U,M, Meitzner K, Ortega-Senovilla H, Graf K, Vetter K, Abou-Dakn M, Herrera E (2011). Differences in the implications of maternal lipids on fetal metabolism and growth between gestational diabetes mellitus and control pregnancies. Diabet. Med. 28: 1053–1059.

[109] Schöndorf T, Maiworm A, Emmison N, Forst T, Pfützner A (2005). Biological background and role of adiponectin as marker for insulin resistance and cardiovascular risk. Clinical Laboratory 51: 489–494.

[110] Seger R and Krebs E.G (1995). The MAPK signaling cascade. FASEB J. 9: 726-735

[111] Shaat N, Groop L (2007). Genetics of gestational diabetes mellitus. Curr Med Chem. 14: 569-83.

[112] Shen Y, Luche R, Wei B, Gordon ML, Diltz CD and Tonks NK (2001). Activation of the Jnk signaling pathway by a dual-specificity phosphatase, JSP-1. PNAS 98: 13613-13618

[113] Shoelson SE, Lee J, Goldfine AB (2006). Inflammation and insulin resistance. J Clin Invest 116 :1793 –1801.

[114] Shoelson S (2002). Invited comment on Ebstein W(1999). On the therapy of diabetes mellitus, in particular on the application of sodium salicylate J Mol Med 80: 618 –619.

[115] Sivan E, Homko CJ, Chen X, Reece EA, Boden G (1999). Effect of insulin on fat metabolism during and after normal pregnancy. Diabetes 48:834–838.

[116] Sorensen RL, Brelje TC (1997). Adaptation of islets of Langerhans to pregnancy: Beta cell growth,enhanced insulin secretion and the role of lactogenic hormones. Hormone metab Res 29: 301-307.

[117] Stefan N, Vozarova B, Funahashi T, Matsuzawa Y, Weyer C, Lindsay RS, Youngren JF, Havel PJ, Pratley RE, Bogardus C, Tataranni PA (2002): Plasma adiponectin concentration is associated with skeletal muscle insulin receptor tyrosine phosphorylation, and low plasma concentration precedes a decrease in whole-body insulin sensitivity in humans. Diabetes 51: 1884 –1888.

[118] Tamura S, Hanada M, Ohnishi M, Katsura K, Sasaki M and Kobayashi T (2002), Regulation of stress-activated protein kinase signaling pathways by protein phosphatases. Eur. J. Biochem; 269: 1060-1066.

[119] Thyfault FP, Hedberg EM, AnchanRM, Thorne OP, Isler CM, Newton ER, Dohm GL, Dde Vente JE (2005). Gestational Diaetes is associated with Depressed Adiponectin levels. Reproductive Sciences 12: 141-145

[120] Tibbles L.A. and Woodgett J.R (1999). The stress activated protein kinase pathways. Cell Mol. Life Sci. 55: 1230-1254.

[121] Tournier C, Dong C, Turner TK, Jones SN, Flavell RA and Davis RJ (2001). MKK7 is an essential component of the JNK signal transduction pathway activated by proinflammatory cytokines. Genes and Dev 15: 1419-1428

[122] Turpin S.M, Lancaster G I, Darby I, Febbraio M A, and Watt M J (2006). Apoptosis in skeletal muscle myotubes is induced by ceramides and is positively related to insulin resistance. Am J. Physiol. Endo. Metab 291:E1341-1350

[123] Veskoukis AS, Tsatsakis AM, Kouretas D (2012). Dietary oxidative stress and antioxidant defense with an emphasis on plant extract administration. Cell Stress Chaperones. 17: 11–21.

[124] Volpe L, Di Cianni G, Lencioni C, Cuccuru I, Benzi L, Del Prato S (2007). Gestational diabetes, inflammation, and late vascular disease. J Endocrinol Invest. 30: 873-879.

[125] Vrachnis N, Belitsos P, Sifakis S, Dafopoulos K, Siristatidis C, Pappa K I, and Iliodromiti Z (2012). Role of Adipokines and Other Inflammatory Mediators in Gestational Diabetes Mellitus and Previous Gestational Diabetes Mellitus Int J Endocrinol. 2012: 549748. Published online April 9, 2012.

[126] Wang B, Jenkins JP,Trayhurn P (2004). Expression and Secretion of inflammation related adipokines by human adipocytes differentiated in cuulture integrated response to TNF-alpha. Am J. Physiol. Endol Metab 288: E731-E740.

[127] Watanabe RM, Black M H, Xiang A H, Allayee H, Lawrence JM, Buchanan TA (2007) Genetics of Gestational Diabetes Mellitus and Type 2 Diabetes. Diabetes Care 30: supplement S134-S140.

[128] Weerakiet S, Srisombut C, Rojanasakul A, Panburana P, Thakkinstian A, Herabutya Y (2004). Prevalence of gestational diabetes mellitus and pregnancy outcomes in Asian women with polycystic ovary syndrome. Gynecol Endocrinol. 19: 134-40.

[129] Weyer C, Funahashi T, Tanaka S, Hotta K, Matsuzawa Y, Pratley RE, Tataranni PA (2001). Hypoadiponectinemia in obesity and type 2 diabetes: close association with insulin resistance and hyperinsulinemia. J Endocrinol Metab 86:1930–1935.

[130] Wiecek A, Adamczak M, Chudek J (2007). Adiponectin—an adipokine with unique metabolic properties. Nephrology Dialysis Transplantation. 22: 981–988.

[131] Winkler G, Cseh K, Baranyi E, Melczer Z, Speer G, Hajos P, Salamon F, Turi Z, Kovacs M, Vargha P, Karadi I (2002): Tumor necrosis factor system and insulin resistance in gestational diabetes. Diabetes Res Clin Pract 56: 93–99.

[132] WHO (2011). Global Strategy on Prevention of Diabetes.

[133] Yudkin J. S, Stehouwer C. D. A., Emeis J. J., and Coppack S. W (1999). C-reactive protein in healthy subjects: associations with obesity, insulin resistance, and endothelial dysfunction: a potential role for cytokines originating from adipose tissue? Arteriosclerosis, Thrombosis, and Vascular Biology 19: 972–978123.

[134] Zavalza-Gómez AB, Anaya-Prado R, Rincón-Sánchez AR, Mora-Martínez JM (2008). Adipokines and insulin resistance during pregnancy. Diabetes Research and Clinical Practice 80: 8–15.

[135] Zhang Y, Proenca R, Maffei M, Barone M, Leopold L, Friedman JM (1994). Positional cloning of the mouse obese gene and its human homologue. Nature 372: 425–432.

[136] Ziegler D (2005). Type 2 diabetes as an inflammatory cardiovascular disorder. Curr Mol Med. 5: 309-22.

Chapter 6

Maternal Hypercholesterolemia in Gestational Diabetes and the Association with Placental Endothelial Dysfunction

A. Leiva, C Diez de Medina, E. Guzmán-Gutierrez,
F. Pardo and L. Sobrevia

Additional information is available at the end of the chapter

http://dx.doi.org/10.5772/55297

1. Introduction

Pregnancy is a physiological condition characterized by a progressive, weeks of gestation-dependent increase in maternal triglycerides (hypertriglyceridemia) and total cholesterol (hypercholesterolemia) [1-4]. In some cases a misadaptation occurs and these levels increase over a physiological range and dyslipidemia is recognized [5]. This condition occurs in some pregnancies coursing without associated pregnancy alterations [i.e., maternal supraphysiological hypercholesterolemia (MSPH)] and in pregnancies coursing with pathologies as preeclampsia and gestational diabetes mellitus (GDM) [3, 5].

GDM is widely associated with endothelial dysfunction of the placenta mainly triggered by hyperinsulinemia, hyperglycemia, and changes in nucleoside extracellular concentration and dyslipidemia associated with this pathology could play a role in this phenomenon since dyslipidemia is a risk factor to develop endothelial dysfunction and atherosclerosis [6]. Additionally, GDM predisposes to an accelerated development of cardiovascular disease (CVD) in adult life and as most of pregnancies with GDM course with elevated dyslipidemia, is feasible found a pathological link between dyslipidemia in GDM pregnancies and development of CVD later in life [6,7].

The hypertrygliceridemia described in GDM is directly related with the fetal macrosomia characteristic of this pathology, and a positive correlation between maternal triglycerides levels and neonatal body weight or fat mass has been found in GDM [7,8].

Even when hypercholesterolemia, described in GDM, is not related with the fetal macrosomia, could be related with fetal endothelial dysfunction and later development of cardiovascular diseases in the adulthood [6].

Although lipid traffic through the placenta is restrictive, a correlation between maternal and fetal blood cholesterol in the first and second trimesters of pregnancy has been established, suggesting that maternal cholesterol level could alter normal development of the fetus [9]. In fact it has been reported that due to altered lipid metabolism in the placenta as a result of high maternal blood cholesterol, atherogenesis, a clinical complication commonly appearing in adults, probably begins in fetal life with similar factors altered at the mother, the fetus and the placenta [9, 10].

In this regard, GDM correlates with placental macro and microvascular endothelial dysfunction, also considered as early marker of atherosclerosis, and neonates from GDM pregnancies have significant increase in the aortic intima-media thickness and higher lipid content, both considered as subclinical markers of atherosclerosis, conditions that will potentially increase the atherosclerotic process later in life [11,12].

Since the lack of information in the literature, nothing is yet available about the potential effect of hypercholesterolemia in GDM pregnancies regarding development of endothelial dysfunction and atherosclerosis in human fetoplacental vasculature [6], however cumulative evidence shows that high levels of blood cholesterol modify the endothelial function in different vascular beds, mostly associated with reduced vascular nitric oxide (NO) bioavailability (i.e. the L-arginine/NO pathway) and elevated oxidative stress leading to reduced vascular reactivity, and then vascular reactivity in children and adults [13].

Several changes caused by hypercholesterolemia could explain these alterations including post-transcriptional down-regulation of cationic amino acid transporters (hCATs)-mediated L-arginine transport [14], reduced NO synthase (NOS) expression [15], reduced expression of tetrahydrobiopterin (BH_4) an NOS cofactor [16], and increased expression and activity of arginases (enzymes that compete by L-arginine with NOS) [17] among others factors that finally leads to reduction of NO synthesis and endothelial dysfunction. Interestingly, these mechanisms have not been evaluated in GDM coursing with hypercholesterolemia [6].

2. Hypercholesterolemia in pregnancy

Several reports show that pregnancy is a physiological condition characterized by a progressive, weeks of gestation-dependent increase (reaching 40-50%) in the maternal blood level of cholesterol [1,2]. This phenomenon is known as maternal physiological hypercholesterolemia in pregnancy (MPH), and is considered to be an adaptive response of the mother to satisfy the high cholesterol demand by the growing fetus [3,4].

In the lack of a consensus and currently available information for general population, a mean value calculated from the reported data in the literature rising to ~247 mg/dl of blood cholesterol could represents a state of MPH (see table 1). When a maternal misadaptation to the cholesterol demand by the fetus occurs, a group of these women develop a pathological condition described as maternal supraphysiological hypercholesterolemia (MSPH) in pregnancy [5]. Unfortunately, the establishment of a cut-point value for this condition is difficult to define because the scare information in the literature regarding this condition. However, a review of the available information allows establish a MSPH condition when the maternal blood cholesterol at term of pregnancy level is over the 90th percentile or establishing a cut-point defined by different authors and based in their findings (Table 1).

With this global lack of information, the prevalence of MSPH in the pregnant population is unknown and could certainly be a consequence of the fact that maternal blood cholesterol level is not routinely evaluated during pregnancy. However, has been reported that the global prevalence for high blood cholesterol level (>200 mg/dl) in non-pregnant women is 40% with a range between 23% (Asia) and 53% (Europe) [18]. Based on this official information from WHO and assuming that pregnancy results in an increase of 40-50% in blood cholesterol [4], it is conceivable that a significant number of women that get pregnant will develop MSPH and who will potentially present an adverse intrauterine condition that could result in facilitating the developing of vascular alterations and atherosclerosis in the growing fetus.

2.1. Cholesterol traffic in pregnancy

Although lipids traffic through the placenta is restrictive and children born from MSPH generally have normal blood cholesterol level [19], a correlation between maternal and fetal blood cholesterol in the first and second trimesters of pregnancy has been established [9,20].

The sources of cholesterol for fetal metabolism along with endogenous production by fetal tissues include transplacental mother-to-fetus transport of cholesterol [9,19,21-26].

The maternal cholesterol must cross two layers of cells to enter in the fetal circulation, the first one are the trophoblast cells and the second one are the endothelial cells [19,27] (Figure 1).

In the maternal circulation the cholesterol is mainly transported in low density (LDL) and high density (HDL) lipoproteins which interacts with their membrane receptors, the LDL receptor (for native LDL (nLDL) and oxidized LDL (ox LDL)), the lectin-like oxidized low-density lipoprotein receptor-1 (LOX-1, for oxLDL), and scavenger receptor class B type I (SR-BI, for HDL and oxLDL) to deliver the cholesterol content into the cell [28,29]. These lipoprotein receptors are expressed in placental cells including trophoblast and endothelial cells [23,30]. Once in the trophoblast cells, the cholesterol may exit cells secreted as lipoprotein or effluxed from the cellular membrane to extracellular acceptors precursors of mature lipoproteins (i.e., apolipoproteins or discoidal phospholipids) [19]. In the next step, this cholesterol is uptake by endothelial cells to be deliver in the fetal circulation, phenomenon where the expression of cholesterol transporters type ATP binding cassette transporter sub-family A member 1 (ABCA1) and sub-family G member 1 (ABCG1) is determinant since these transporters participate in the efflux of cholesterol to nascent fetal lipoproteins [26,31]. In this scenery the phospholipid transporter protein (PLTP) also participate in the formation of fetal HDL (fHDL) contributing with the efflux of phospholipids to nascent fHDL [26] (Figure 1).

Studied population (n)	Blood cholesterol (mg/dl)		Ref.
	MPH	Cut-point for MSPH	
USA (29)	251	318	[5]
USA (142)	260	300	[157]
USA (553)	250	300	[158]
Canada (59)	248	290	[24]
Mexico (130)	189	-	[159]
Argentina (101)	244	-	[160]
Chile (86)	263	280	[unpublished]
UK (8)	289	-	[161]
UK (40)	315	-	[162]
UK (114)	273	-	[163]
UK (118)	246	-	[163]
UK (178)	264	-	[164]
Italy (82)	-	281	[9]
Italy (156)	-	280	[21]
Italy (72)	205	280	[165]
Italy (22)	286	-	[1]
Norway (12.573)	211	-	[166]
France (73)	242	-	[167]
Germany (150)	253	-	[168]
Spain (45)	225	-	[143]
Spain (66)	259	-	[169]
Portugal (67)	285	-	[170]
Finland (22)	274	-	[171]
Japan (19)	280	-	[172]
China (20)	184	-	[173]
Pakistan (45)	209	-	[174]
Nigeria (222)	204	-	[175]
Tunisia (30)	222	-	[176]
Mean	247		

The values correspond to the third trimester of pregnancy. MPH: maternal physiological and hypercholesterolemia, MSPH: maternal supraphysiological hypercholesterolemia.

Table 1. Maternal total cholesterol in MPH and MSPH pregnancies.

http://dx.doi.org/10.5772/55297

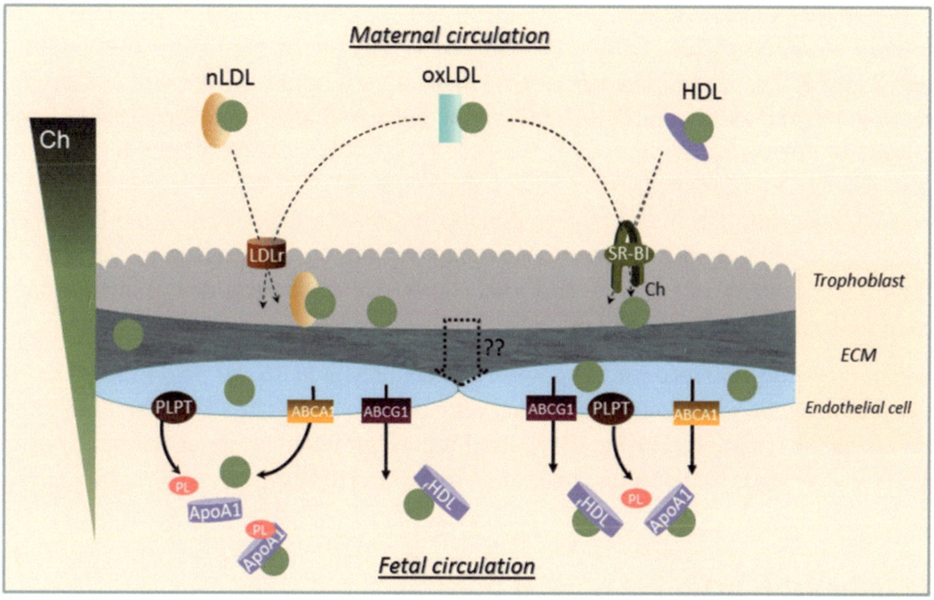

Figure 1. Mother-to-fetus transport of maternal cholesterol. In the maternal circulation (higher levels of plasma cholesterol) the cholesterol (Ch) is mainly transported in low density lipoproteins (LDL) (natives, nLDL and oxidized, oxLDL) and high density lipoproteins (HDL) lipoproteins and delivered into the trophoblast by LDL receptor (LDL-r) and scavenger receptor class B type I (SR-BI). The cholesterol deliver to extracellular matrix (ECM) and is uptake by endothelial cells through unknown mechanisms to finally, be delivered to the fetal circulation by the of cholesterol transporters type ATP binding cassette transporter sub-family A member 1 (ABCA1) and sub-family G member 1 (ABCG1), which together with phospholipid (PL)-transfer protein (PLPT) contribute with the assembly of fetal lipoproteins. In fetal circulation (lower levels of plasma cholesterol) cholesterol is deliver to acceptors as ApoAI and nascent fetal HDL (fHDL).

Thus the mother-*to*-fetus transport of cholesterol seems to be a controlled process that is crucial in fetal development; however the effect of a supraphysiological level of maternal cholesterol will modify the traffic of cholesterol increasing the risk of developing fetal vascular anomalies such as those seen in atherosclerosis [31].

2.2. Consequences of MSPH in the fetus

Studies in aortas from spontaneously aborted human fetuses and premature newborns (24-30 weeks of gestation) demonstrate that offspring from mothers with MSPH in pregnancy exhibit more and larger aortic lesion which were positive for almost one marker of atherosclerosis among the presence of macrophages and foam cell, LDL, oxLDL and oxidation-specific epitopes [9]. These data were additionally supported by another autopsy study that determined that children (1-13 years old) of mothers with MSPH in pregnancy exhibit faster progression of atherosclerotic lesions [21].

At present, the effect of MSPH have been evaluated as atherosclerosis in fetal arteries but the vascular effects of MSPH could be determined in placental vessels since its cells are indirectly exposed to maternal cholesterol (see section *Cholesterol traffic in pregnancy*). Interestingly, it has been shown that MSPH is associated with increased expression of placental genes related to cholesterol metabolism (i.e. fatty acid synthase (FAS), sterol regulatory element-binding protein 2 (SREBP2)), thus exposing the fetus to an altered lipid environment and eventually promoting vascular alterations [24]. Additionally, increased level of maternal cholesterol and LDL leads to down-regulation of LDL receptor expression in whole placenta homogenized without changes in the expression of HDL receptor (SR-BI) [32], suggesting that the increase in the LDL concentration in the maternal blood induce the regulation of the LDL receptor expression. Interestingly these alterations are not related with changes in the newborn lipid levels, in fact normal levels of LDL and total cholesterol are determined at birth in the fetal blood of newborns from mothers with MSPH.

These data provide evidence for the potential effect of MSPH on the placenta and its consequences for the fetus where vascular lesion progression is triggered. However, even knowing this available information nothing is reported regarding whether abnormal maternal blood cholesterol level leads to placental vascular dysfunction [10,33].

3. Endothelial function in normal pregnancies

The placenta is a physical and metabolic barrier between the fetal and maternal circulation. The normal development and function of the placenta and the umbilical cord are crucial to sustain the adequate fetal development and growth [34]. The human fetoplacental circulation under physiological conditions exhibits a high blood flow and low vascular resistance [35]. Since it lacks of autonomic innervation [36] the equilibrium between the synthesis, release and bioavailability of vasoconstrictors and vasodilators circulating and locally released, such as NO and adenosine, are crucial to maintain the control of fetoplacental hemodynamics [37,38]. In a physiological context, different pathologies of pregnancy such as GDM [38,39], intrauterine growth restriction (IUGR) [40] or preeclampsia [41], exhibits altered synthesis and/or bioavailability of NO leading to changes in blood flow of the human placenta thus limiting fetal growth and development [37,38,42]. These conditions produce an imbalance or loss of essential endothelial functions leading to altered blood flow in the fetoplacental unit mainly associated with altered NO synthesis and membrane transport of the semi-essential cationic amino acid L-arginine, i.e., the 'endothelial L-arginine/NO pathway' (Figure 2) [35,42,43].

3.1. Endothelial L-arginine/NO signaling pathway

Synthesis of NO requires active NOS, a group of enzymes conformed by, at least, three isoforms, i.e., neuronal NOS (nNOS or type 1), inducible NOS (iNOS or type 2) and endothelial NOS (eNOS or type 3), of which mainly eNOS is expressed in endothelial cells [43,44]. The NO diffuses from endothelium to vascular smooth muscle cells leading to cyclic GMP (cGMP)-dependent vasodilatation [45].

Activity of NOS may depend on the ability of endothelial cells to take up its specific substrate L-arginine via a variety of membrane transport systems [42,43,46,47]. L-Arginine is taken up into the endothelial cells through the membrane transport systems y^+ (cationic amino acid

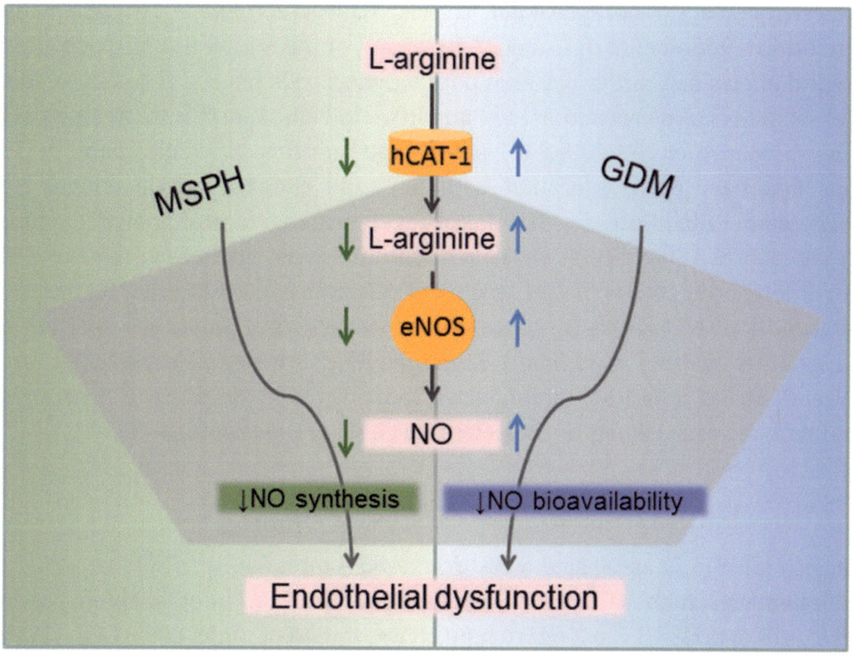

Figure 2. Endothelial L-Arginine/NO pathway regulation by GDM and MSPH. In human endothelial cells L-arginine is mainly taken up via cationic amino acid transporter 1 (hCAT-1). Then, L-arginine is metabolized in nitric oxide (NO) and L-citrulline by endothelial NO synthase (eNOS). In GDM is described an increase (blue up arrows) in the elements in L-Arginine/NO pathway, but with a decrease in NO bioavailability leading endothelial dysfunction. As seen in other vascular beds, MSPH leads to decreased (green down arrows) hCAT-1 and eNOS expression; and NO synthesis leading also to endothelial dysfunction.

transporters family, CATs), y^+L (very high affinity transporters), $b^{0,+}$ and $B^{0,+}$ (Na^+-independent and dependent, respectively) [48,49,50]. CATs is a family of membrane transporters with at least 5 isoforms identified in human tissues, i.e., human CAT-1 (hCAT-1), hCAT-2A, hCAT-2B, hCAT-3 and hCAT-4 [43,51]. In endothelial cells from the human placenta such as human umbilical vein endothelial cells (HUVEC) and human placental microvascular endothelial cells (hPMEC), only hCAT-1 and hCAT-2B isoforms like transport have been identified, the first exhibiting low-capacity and high-affinity, and the second exhibiting higher-capacity and lower-affinity [41,51]. Moreover, eNOS activity seems to depend on the ability of these cells to take up L-arginine mainly via hCAT-1 and/or hCAT-2B [40, 33, 52]. Interestingly in pathological conditions such as GDM the L-arginine/NO pathway is highly up-regulated in HUVEC [6, 39, 53, 54] (Figure 2).

4. Hypercholesterolemia and endothelial L-arginine/NO pathway

Endothelial dysfunction and reduced NO seems are considered early markers in the development of cardiovascular disease [55-58]. Thus, studies designed to evaluate the impact of hypercholesterolemia (in non-placental vessels) have determined that this pathological condition induces endothelial dysfunction in vessels of the macro and microcirculation, but the biological effects may differ between both vascular beds [59-60]. It has been shown that high levels of total cholesterol and oxLDL impair endothelial function increasing the production of the vasoconstrictor endothelin-1 [61-62] and reducing NO bioavailability [13,63-67], alterations that have been associated with impaired endothelium-dependent relaxation [68-73]. Therefore, alterations in cholesterol levels leading to endothelial dysfunction in different vascular beds have been associated with molecular changes in the expression and activity of different component of the L-arginine/NO pathway, thus decreasing the production or bioavailability of NO (Table 2). However, no studies have addressed whether elevated maternal blood cholesterol modulate L-arginine/NO pathway and endothelial function in placental endothelial cells form pregnancies coursing with MSPH or pregnancy diseases associated with increased levels of cholesterol as GDM or preeclampsia [12,35].

4.1. eNOS expression and activity in hypercholesterolemia

Hypercholesterolemia is associated with decreased expression of eNOS in aortic rings of hypercholesterolemic rabbits [58] and in human saphenous vein endothelial cell, porcine aortic endothelial cells and HUVEC expose to high concentration of nLDL or ox-LDL [15,75,76], an effect that is reversed by restitution of normal blood cholesterol level (e.g., with the use of statins). The mechanism behind this effect of hypercholesterolemia on eNOS expression is not well understood and few studies have proposed a time- and concentration-dependent decrease in eNOS mRNA level involving transcriptional inhibition and reduced mRNA stability (i.e., reducing eNOS mRNA half-life) [15,75,76].

Additionally to down regulation of eNOS expression, high levels of cholesterol are also associated with changes in eNOS cellular localization and function, a phenomenon related with up-regulation of the protein caveolin [77-83]. In the endothelial cell eNOS targets to caveolae [70,71] where it is functionally inhibited by binding to caveolin [84-87]. Optimal eNOS activity occurs when the eNOS-caveolin complex interaction is disrupted by calcium-calmodulin binding to eNOS-caveolin [87]. It has been shown that caveolin expression is regulated by cholesterol increasing eNOS-caveolin complex formation, and diminishing NO production [88-90].

4.2. Asymmetrical dimethylarginine (ADMA) availability in hypercholesterolemia

ADMA, an arginine metabolite proposed as endogenous inhibitor of eNOS [91-95], is increased in hypercholesterolemic monkeys [92] and in human endothelial cells incubated with high concentration of nLDL and oxLDL [96]. The mechanisms involved in this phenomenon are the up-regulation of the expression of protein arginine N-methyl transferases (PRMTs), which are involved in the synthesis of ADMA and decreased activity of dimethylarginine dimethylaminohydrolase (DDAH), an enzyme responsible of ADMA degradation [78,82,83]. Moreover, the regulation of ADMA is relevant in the atherogenic process and extensive data have shown a good correlation between plasmatic levels of ADMA and the presence of atherosclerosis [92].

Element	Gestational Diabetes Mellitus			Non-pregnancy Hypercholesterolemia		
	Cell type	Effect	References	Cell type	Effect	References
hCATs expression	HUVEC	Increased	[43]	EAhy926	Increased	[113]
				rAR	Increased	[114]
hCATs activity	HUVEC	Increased	[43]	EAhy926	Increased	[113]
				rAR	Reduced	[14]
				bAEC	Reduced	[111]
				pAEC	Reduced	[74]
				HUVEC	Unaltered	[109]
				HUVEC	Unaltered	[110]
eNOS expression	HUVEC	Increased	[28,43]	hSVEC	Reduced	[15]
	hPT	Increased	[177]	rbAS	Increased	[75]
				rbAS	Reduced	[152]
				HUVEC	Reduced	[76]
				pAEC	Reduced	[180]
eNOS activity	HUVEC	Increased	[28,29,43]	hSVEC	Reduced	[15]
	hVT	Unaltered	[178]	rbAS	Reduced	[152]
				HUVEC	Reduced	[76]
				pAEC	Reduced	[74]
				rAC	Reduced	[181]
NO level	HUVEC	Increased	[179]	hSVEC	Reduced	[15]
Arginase I				hPBMC	Increased	[182]
Arginase II				hAEC	Increased	[17,114,115]
				mAEC	Increased	[114,115]

hCATs, human cationic amino acid transporters; eNOS, endothelial nitric oxide synthase; NO, nitric oxide; HUVEC, human umbilical vein endothelial cell; hPT, human placental tissue; hVT, human villous tissue; EAhy 926, human endothelial cell line EAhy 926; rAR, rat aortic ring; bAEC, bovine aortic endothelial cell; pAEC, porcine aortic endothelial cell; hSVEC, human saphenous vein endothelial cell; rbAS, rabbit aortic segment; rAC, rat aortic cell; hPBMC, peripheral blood mononuclear cells; hAEC, human aortic endothelial cell; mAEC, mouse aortic endothelial cell. Table modified from reference 6.

Table 2. Effect of GDM and hypercholesterolemia on endothelial L-Arginine/NO pathway.

Thus, this is a different way by which increased levels of cholesterol leads to a reduction in NO synthesis.

4.3. Tetrahydrobiopterin (BH_4) availability in hypercholesterolemia

A reduced expression of the eNOS cofactor BH_4 leads to deficient activation (or even uncoupling) of eNOS, a phenomenon characterized by eNOS-reduction of molecular oxygen by a no longer coupled L-arginine oxidative mechanism resulting in generation of superoxide anion rather than NO [98]. This phenomenon contributes to vascular oxidative stress and endothelial damage and dysfunction [16]. Hypercholesterolemic mice and rabbit exhibit reduced level of BH_4 in the aorta and myocardium [99,100], a phenomenon related with endothelial dysfunction and major progression of atherosclerosis. Additionally, it has been demonstrated that BH_4 supplementation improves the endothelial function in hypercholesterolemic patients [101,102], suggesting that this cofactor is reduced in this pathological condition. Endothelial cells from the human placenta vasculature express functional BH_4 which is reduced with the progress of pregnancy by a mechanism involving lower activity of guanosine triphosphate cyclohydrolase I (GTPCH) and 6-pyruvoyl tetrahydropterin synthase (PTPS), key enzymes involved in BH_4 synthesis [103,104]. Alternatively, in other cell types, a reduced level of BH_4 dependent of down-regulation of GTPCH expression has been associated with hypercholesterolemia in rat macrophages and smooth muscle cells [105,106].

4.4. L-Arginine transport in hypercholesterolemia

Decreased bioavailability of L-arginine could result from reduced expression and/or altered cellular localization of hCATs, as reported for hCAT-1 and potentially hCAT-2B in HUVEC [53,54,107,108]. Interestingly, it was initially shown that hCAT-1–like transport was unaltered by oxLDL in HUVEC cultures [109,110]. However, no kinetic parameters were addressed in these studies opening the possibility that L-arginine transport at a unique fixed concentration of this amino acid (100 μM) [109] could be insensible to oxLDL, or that a long period of incubation for L-arginine uptake (1-24 hours) [110] will not be a condition close to initial velocity for transport, something required for this type of analysis [49,51]. Additional studies in other types of endothelial cells show that LDL (native or oxLDL) reduces L-arginine transport in aortic endothelium from hypercholesterolemic rats, involving protein kinase C [14]; and bovine aortic endothelium where a maximal transport capacity (V_{max}/K_m) [49] is reduced [111,112]. Interestingly, human aortic endothelial cells exposed to nLDL/oXLDL exhibit decreased intracellular content of L-arginine, a phenomenon explained as resulting from post-translational down-regulation of CAT1 and increased CAT1 internalization [102]. In addition, and highlighting the involvement of L-arginine transport in placental vascular reactivity, recent studies suggest that L-arginine transport mediated by hCAT-1 will be a mechanism limiting human placental vascular reactivity since reduced transport (by the use of *N*-ethylmaleimide) or cross-inhibition (by L-lysine) of hCATs leads to reduced insulin-induced dilatation of human umbilical vein rings from normal pregnancies [54].

4.5. Arginases expression in hypercholesterolemia

Up-regulation of arginases (isoforms I and II) is another mechanism by which NO synthesis is proposed to be reduced leading to placental endothelial dysfunction. Arginases are enzyme competing by L-arginine with eNOS [17,114,115], favoring conversion of L-arginine into L-ornithine and urea. Therefore, an increase in arginases activity will limit the availability of L-arginine to be metabolized by eNOS for NO synthesis. Interestingly, a link between hypercholesterolemia and arginase I and II expression has been demonstrated in mice [115] and in human aortic endothelial cells [116] where oxLDL induces an overexpression of arginases and a reduction of total eNOS protein abundance associated with lower NO production [114], mostly by the interaction with LOX-1 receptor and the activation of the small GTPase RhoA and Rho A kinase (ROCK) signaling pathway [17]. Interestingly, the reduction of arginases activity caused by statins in hypercholesterolemic subjects improves the endothelial function [117]. These findings show that arginases could play a role in the modulation of endothelial function, most likely regarding NO synthesis by competing for L-arginine with eNOS.

5. Gestational diabetes mellitus

GDM is a syndrome characterized by glucose intolerance with onset or first recognition during pregnancy [118-120]. Clinical manifestations of GDM have been attributed mainly to the condition of hyperglycemia, hyperlipidemia, hyperinsulinemia, and fetoplacental endothelial dysfunction [34,37,119,121,123]. GDM is also associated with abnormal fetal development and perinatal complications, such as macrosomia, neonatal hypoglycemia, and neurological disorders [121]. This syndrome occurs with a high incidence, depending on diagnostic criteria used, ranging between 5 and 15% of pregnant women in developing [124,125] and developed countries [120,126-128].

Altered vascular reactivity is a characteristic of GDM and is due to endothelial dysfunction at the micro and macro fetoplacental vasculature [34,37,129-134].

Even when hyperglycaemia is the principal factor leading to endothelial dysfunction, other factors are involved including hyperinsulinemia and the extracellular nucleoside adenosine level [39,133,134]. Since GDM is associated with MSPH, this factor could also contribute with this phenomenon although the effect is actually unknown.

5.1. Endothelial function in GDM and L-arginine/NO pathway

It has been reported that the NO level in the human umbilical vein blood is increased in GDM [127] and that in HUVEC from GDM the synthesis of NO is increased [39,53, 135, 136]. These findings were associated with a constitutive increase in the number of copies for eNOS mRNA, as well as increased eNOS protein level and activity. Other studies show that in HUVEC isolated from GDM the L-arginine transport is increased due to higher maximal velocity (V_{max}) for transport, most likely resulting from increased expression of hCAT-1 [53,133]. Even when the synthesis of NO is increased in GDM cells, the bioavailability of this vasodilator is reduced leading to an state of endothelial dysfunction [6,34,39, 123] (Figure 2). Thus, the vascular reactivity of umbilical vein rings from GDM is lower compare with rings from normal pregnancies [39]. This phenomenon has been suggested to result from a less reactive umbilical vein due to a tonic and basal increased state of vasodilation by over-release and/or accumulation of adenosine, a nucleoside that induce vascular relaxation, in the umbilical vein blood [39].

6. Dyslipidemia in GDM

GDM is a pathological condition also characterized by maternal dyslipidemia, alterations that affect directly the fetal development and growth [123].

Dyslipidemia is defined as elevated levels of triglycerides (hypertriglyceridemia) and total blood cholesterol (hypercholesterolemia) including increased LDL and reduced HDL cholesterol [137]. Dyslipidemia is recognized as the main risk factor for development of CVD [137,139]. Additionally, GDM has also been established as a significant risk factor to fetal programming of metabolic syndrome [140-142] and thus predisposing to accelerate the development of CVD in the adult life [141-146].

Interestingly, most of pregnancies that develop GDM course with dyslipidemia [7,24,147] (Table 3) and thus could be feasible to found a pathologic link between dyslipidemia in pregnancies with GDM and the development of CVD later in life.

GDM is related with fetal macrosomia and endothelial dysfunction and interestingly both characteristic could be related with the associated dyslipidemia. The association between dyslipidemia and macrosomia regards hypertriglyceridemia more than hypercholesterolemia; in fact, a positive correlation between maternal triglycerides and neonatal body weight or fat mass has been found in GDM [7,141,142]. In the other hand, hypercholesterolemia could contribute with the endothelial dysfunction described in the pathology [6,142,149]. Thus GDM could play a role in the fetal programming of adult CVD not only by the classical alterations mainly triggered by hyperinsulinemia, hyperglycaemia and changes in nucleoside extracellular concentration, but also by hypercholesterolemia associated with this pathology [6,142,149]. However, no studies have addressed whether elevated maternal blood cholesterol in GDM modulate endothelial function in placental endothelial cells [33].

6.1. Cholesterol metabolism in GDM

The increased levels of maternal cholesterol in GDM (Table 3) are related with alterations in the expression of proteins involved in lipid and cholesterol homeostasis [24,150,151].

Although MSPH is associated with decreased expression of LDL receptor in the placenta, the effect of GDM-associated dyslipidemia on lipoprotein receptors expression is unknown [24,32]. A study of microarray profile determined changes in the expression of multiple genes involved in lipid and cholesterol metabolism in placental tissue of pregnancies coursing with GDM. These genes include the fatty acid coenzyme A ligase, long chain 2, 3 and 4 (FACL2,3,4) that catalyze the conversion of fatty acids into fatty acyl-CoA esters (precursors for the synthesis of triglycerides, cholesterol, and membrane phospholipids), additionally 3-hydroxy-3-methylglutaryl-Coenzyme A reductase (HMGCR), 3-hydroxy-3-methylglutaryl-

	1°trimester	2°trimester	3°trimester	Reference
TG	101*	142*	187*	[147]
(mg/dl)		286*	271*	[183]
			226*	[184]
			260*	[185]
			268	[24]
			220	[158]
			203	[186]
		214		[187]
Ch	203*	226*	281*	[147]
(mg/dl)		241	224	[183]
			242	[184]
			267	[24]
			197	[158]
			243	[185]
		246		[187]
LDL		145	130	[183]
(mg/dl)		129		[187]
			130	[184]
			148†	[185]
			143	[24]
			197	[158]

Values of cholesterol (Ch) and triglycerides (TG) in GDM pregnancies were compared with those of normal pregnancy. *: level increased compared with a control group without GDM. †: level decreases compared with a control group without GDM. LDL: low-density lipoprotein.

Table 3. Maternal lipids levels GDM pregnancies.

Coenzyme A synthase (HMGCS 1) among other genes involved in the novo synthesis of cholesterol were also regulated [150] and even when in this study the level of cholesterol were not determined among normal and GDM pregnancies, these data suggest that GDM leads to changes in genes related with cholesterol metabolism in the placenta. Previously was described that MSPH associates with increased expression of FAS and SREBP2 in the placenta, while the effect in FAS was observed also in placental cells from GDM without changes in SREBP2 expression [24].

These data suggest that both MSPH and GDM associates with changes in key element in the lipids metabolism, however, if MSPH potentiate the effect of GDM over theses parameters is unknown [6].

Another lipid modulator modified by GDM in placental cells is PLTP, a key protein involved in the metabolism of fetal HDL. PLTP is expressed in endothelial cells of the placental vasculature and is regulated as ABCA1 and ABCG1 by liver X receptor (LXR) nuclear receptors [26,152,153]. Interestingly diabetes leads to increased levels of the principal ligand of LXR, the oxysterols [154] and GDM associates with up-regulation of PLTP in endothelial cells of the placenta [151] mainly due to the hyperinsulinemia and hyperglycaemia related with GDM. The increased expression of PLTP could be a key phenomenon associated with the increased concentration of HDL described in newborns from GDM [11,151]. Additionally, the increased expression of PLTP in placental endothelial cells could affect the maternal to fetal cholesterol transport, a phenomenon not yet evaluated and potential worsen by conditions as MSPH where the mother-*to*-fetus cholesterol transport may be altered almost in the first months of pregnancies when the levels maternal cholesterol correlates with the fetal ones [9].

6.2. Hypercholesterolemia in GDM and endothelial dysfunction

As was previously discussed, physiological increase in the levels of maternal cholesterol is considered to be an adaptive response of the mother to satisfy the high lipids demand by the growing fetus. The misadaptation to this condition leads to develop MSPH a phenomenon associated with the earlier development of fetal atherosclerosis and with reduced endothelial function of the umbilical vein [6].

Additionally and regarding with the development of atherosclerosis, it is recognized that GDM correlates with endothelial dysfunction [34,39] and neonates of pregnancies coursing with GDM have significant increase in aortic and umbilical artery intima-media thickness (IMT) and higher lipid content, both markers of subclinical atherosclerosis that could increase the atherosclerotic process later in life [12,155,156].

The effect of GDM in the aortic IMT of newborns was assayed and an increased intimal-medial ratio was determined. Interestingly the IMT was evaluated in newborns of pregnancies coursing with GDM and increased levels of total cholesterol and LDL compared with the control group [12]. Thereby may be possible to found a potential effect of MSPH in this phenomenon. Similar findings were found in fetus in the lasts weeks of gestation where the IMT was evaluated in umbilical artery, where umbilical IMT was increased in arteries from GDM pregnancies, however the potential effect of maternal cholesterol was not evaluated [156].

http://dx.doi.org/10.5772/55297

Unfortunately, nothing is yet available regarding the potential effects of MSPH in pregnancies coursing with GDM on the development of endothelial dysfunction and atherosclerosis in placental and eventually in fetal vessels at birth, a phenomenon that could leads to a potentiation of GDM-associated fetoplacental endothelial dysfunction.

7. Concluding remarks

MSPH is a risk factor promoting the development of atherosclerosis in the growing fetus and in the children, however the effects of this condition in fetoplacental endothelium is unknown even when increased levels of maternal cholesterol could lead to alterations in the hCAT-mediated L-arginine transport and eNOS-synthesis of NO (i.e., the endothelial L-arginine/NO signaling pathway) such as occurs in other vascular beds exposed to high cholesterol levels.

GDM is a condition that course with alterations of the L-arginine/NO signaling pathway in the human fetoplacental vasculature, phenomenon resulting in abnormal bioavailability of NO leading to altered vascular reactivity and changes in umbilical vessels blood flow with consequences in the fetal growth and development.

Interestingly, some pregnancies coursing with GDM associates with MSPH and the possibility that the observed fetoplacental endothelial dysfunction results from a potentiation of the classical factor associated with GDM and the increased levels of cholesterol is likely.

Further studies are required to elucidate whether pregnancies coursing with GDM and MSPH have different effect in placental endothelial function compare with those coursing with GDM and normal levels of maternal cholesterol because it could be possible find a different mechanism involved in both cases.

This may contribute to understand the mechanisms related with the vascular dysfunction associated with GDM and allow establishing a better knowledge based- management of the mother and the newborn.

Acknowledgements

We are thankful to the personnel at the Hospital Clínico Pontificia Universidad Católica de Chile labour ward for their support in the supply of placentas. This research was funded by Fondo Nacional de Desarrollo Científico y Tecnológico (FONDECYT 1110977, 11110059, 3130583), Programa de Investigación Interdisciplinario (PIA) from Comisión Nacional de Investigación en Ciencia y Tecnología (CONICYT, Anillos ACT-73) (Chile) and CONICYT Ayuda de Tesis (CONICYT AT-24120944). EG-G holds a CONICYT-PhD (Chile) fellowship. FP was the recipient of a postdoctoral position (CONICYT PIA Anillos ACT-73 postdoctoral research associate at CMPL, Pontificia Universidad Católica de Chile (PUC)). CDM was the recipient of an undergraduate research position (CONICYT PIA Anillos ACT-73 undergraduate researcher at CMPL, PUC).

Author details

A. Leiva*, C Diez de Medina, E. Guzmán-Gutierrez, F. Pardo and L. Sobrevia

*Address all correspondence to: aaleiva@puc.cl, sobrevia@med.puc.cl

Cellular and Molecular Physiology Laboratory (CMPL), Division of Obstetrics and Gynecology, Faculty of Medicine, School of Medicine, Pontificia Universidad Católica de Chile, Chile

References

[1] Brizzi P, Tonolo G, Esposito F, Puddu L, Dessole S, Maioli M, et al. (1999) Lipoprotein metabolism during normal pregnancy. American journal of obstetrics and gynecology 181: 430-434.

[2] Avis HJ, Hutten BA, Twickler MT, Kastelein JJ, van der Post JA, Stalenhoef AF, et al. (2009) Pregnancy in women suffering from familial hypercholesterolemia: a harmful period for both mother and newborn? Current opinion in lipidology 20:484-490.

[3] Schaefer-Graf UM, Meitzner K, Ortega-Senovilla H, Graf K, Vetter K, Abou-Dakn M, et al. (2011) Differences in the implications of maternal lipids on fetal metabolism and growth between gestational diabetes mellitus and control pregnancies. Diabetic medicine 28:1053-1059.

[4] Basaran A (2009) Pregnancy-induced hyperlipoproteinemia: review of the literature. Reproductive sciences 16:431-437.

[5] Montes A, Walden CE, Knopp RH, Cheung M, Chapman MB, Albers JJ (1984) Physiologic and supraphysiologic increases in lipoprotein lipids and apoproteins in late pregnancy and postpartum. Possible markers for the diagnosis of "prelipemia". Arteriosclerosis 4:407-417.

[6] Leiva A, Pardo F, Ramirez MA, Farias M, Casanello P, Sobrevia L (2011) Fetoplacental vascular endothelial dysfunction as an early phenomenon in the programming of human adult diseases in subjects born from gestational diabetes mellitus or obesity in pregnancy. Experimental diabetes research 2011:349286.

[7] Herrera E, Ortega-Senovilla H (2010) Disturbances in lipid metabolism in diabetic pregnancy - Are these the cause of the problem? Best practice and research. Clinical endocrinology & metabolism 24:515-525.

[8] Son GH, Kwon JY, Kim YH, Park YW (2010)Maternal serum triglycerides as predictive factors for large-for-gestational age newborns in women with gestational diabetes mellitus. Acta Obstetrics and Gynecology Scandinav 89:700-704.

[9] Napoli C, D'Armiento FP, Mancini FP, Postiglione A, Witztum JL, Palumbo G, et al. (1997) Fatty streak formation occurs in human fetal aortas and is greatly enhanced by maternal hypercholesterolemia. Intimal accumulation of low density lipoprotein and its oxidation precede monocyte recruitment into early atherosclerotic lesions. The Journal of clinical investigation 100:2680-2690.

[10] Palinski W, Napoli C (2002) The fetal origins of atherosclerosis: maternal hypercholesterolemia, and cholesterol-lowering or antioxidant treatment during pregnancy influence in utero programming and postnatal susceptibility to atherogenesis. FASEB journal 16:1348-1360.

[11] Merzouk H, Madani S, Prost J, Loukidi B, Meghelli-Bouchenak M, Belleville J (1999) Changes in serum lipid and lipoprotein concentrations and compositions at birth and after 1 month of life in macrosomic infants of insulin-dependent diabetic mothers. European Journal of Pediatrics 158:750-756.

[12] Koklu E, Akcakus M, Kurtoglu S, Koklu S, Yikilmaz A, Coskun A, et al. (2007) Aortic intima-media thickness and lipid profile in macrosomic newborns. European Journal of Pediatrics 166:333-338.

[13] Landmesser U, Hornig B, Drexler H (2000) Endothelial dysfunction in hypercholesterolemia: mechanisms, pathophysiological importance, and therapeutic interventions. Seminars in Thrombosis and Hemostasis 26:529-537.

[14] Schwartz IF, Ingbir M, Chernichovski T, Reshef R, Chernin G, Litvak A, et al. (2007) Arginine uptake is attenuated, through post-translational regulation of cationic amino acid transporter-1, in hyperlipidemic rats. Atherosclerosis 194:357-363.

[15] Liao JK, Shin WS, Lee WY, Clark SL (1995) Oxidized low-density lipoprotein decreases the expression of endothelial nitric oxide synthase. The Journal of Biological Chemistry 270:319-324.

[16] Alp NJ, Channon KM (2004) Regulation of endothelial nitric oxide synthase by tetrahydrobiopterin in vascular disease. Arteriosclerosis, Thrombosis, and Vascular Biology 24:413-420.

[17] Ryoo S, Lemmon CA, Soucy KG, Gupta G, White AR, Nyhan D, et al. (2006) Oxidized low-density lipoprotein-dependent endothelial arginase II activation contributes to impaired nitric oxide signaling. Circulation research 99:951-960.

[18] World Health Organization (2010) Global status report on non-communicable diseases 1:9-31

[19] Woollett LA (2011) Review: Transport of maternal cholesterol to the fetal circulation. Placenta 32:S218-S221.

[20] Badruddin SH, Lalani R, Khurshid M, Molla A, Qureshi R, Khan MA (1990) Serum cholesterol in neonates and their mothers. A pilot study. Journal of Pakistan Medical Association 40:108-109.

[21] Napoli C, Glass CK, Witztum JL, Deutsch R, D'Armiento FP, Palinski W (1999) Influence of maternal hypercholesterolaemia during pregnancy on progression of early atherosclerotic lesions in childhood: Fate of Early Lesions in Children (FELIC) study. Lancet 354:1234-1241.

[22] Battaile KP, Steiner RD (2000) Smith-Lemli-Opitz syndrome: the first malformation syndrome associated with defective cholesterol synthesis. Molecular genetics and metabolism 71:154-162.

[23] Wadsack C, Hammer A, Levak-Frank S, Desoye G, Kozarsky KF, Hirschmugl B, et al. (2003) Selective cholesteryl ester uptake from high density lipoprotein by human first trimester and term villous trophoblast cells. Placenta 24:131-143.

[24] Marseille-Tremblay C, Ethier-Chiasson M, Forest JC, Giguere Y, Masse A, Mounier C, et al. (2008) Impact of maternal circulating cholesterol and gestational diabetes mellitus on lipid metabolism in human term placenta. Molecular reproduction and development 75:1054-1062.

[25] Jenkins KT, Merkens LS, Tubb MR, Myatt L, Davidson WS, Steiner RD, et al. (2008) Enhanced placental cholesterol efflux by fetal HDL in Smith-Lemli-Opitz syndrome. Molecular genetics and metabolism 94:240-247.

[26] Stefulj J, Panzenboeck U, Becker T, Hirschmugl B, Schweinzer C, Lang I, et al. (2009) Human endothelial cells of the placental barrier efficiently deliver cholesterol to the fetal circulation via ABCA1 and ABCG1. Circulation research 104:600-608.

[27] Desoye G, Gauster M, Wadsack C. (2011) Placental transport in pregnancy pathologies. American Journal of Clinical Nutrition. 94:S1896-S1902.

[28] Chen M, Masaki T, Sawamura T (2002) LOX-1, the receptor for oxidized low-density lipoprotein identified from endothelial cells: implications in endothelial dysfunction and atherosclerosis. 95:89-100.

[29] Mineo C, Deguchi H, Griffin JH, Shaul PW (2006) Endothelial and antithrombotic actions of HDL. Pharmacology and Therapeutics 98:1352-1364.

[30] Marsche G, Levak-Frank S, Quehenberger O, Heller R, Sattler W, Malle E (2001) Identification of the human analog of SR-BI and LOX-1 as receptors for hypochlorite-modified high density lipoprotein on human umbilical venous endothelial cells. FASEB journal 15:1095-1097.

[31] Palinski W, Nicolaides E, Liguori A, Napoli C (2009) Influence of maternal dysmetabolic conditions during pregnancy on cardiovascular disease. Journal of cardiovascular translational research 2:277-285.

[32] Ethier-Chiasson M, Duchesne A, Forest JC, Giguere Y, Masse A, Mounier C, et al. (2007) Influence of maternal lipid profile on placental protein expression of LDLr and SR-BI. Biochemical and biophysical research communications 359:8-14.

[33] Joles JA (2011) Crossing borders: linking environmental and genetic developmental factors. Micricirculation 18:298-303.

[34] Sobrevia L, Abarzua F, Nien JK, Salomon C, Westermeier F, Puebla C, et al. (2011) Review: Differential placental macrovascular and microvascular endothelial dysfunction in gestational diabetes. Placenta 32:S159-S164.

[35] Myatt L (2010) Review: Reactive oxygen and nitrogen species and functional adaptation of the placenta. Placenta 31:S66-S69.

[36] Marzioni D, Tamagnone L, Capparuccia L, Marchini C, Amici A, Todros T, et al. (2004) Restricted innervation of uterus and placenta during pregnancy: evidence for a role of the repelling signal Semaphorin 3A. Developmental Dynamics 231:839-848.

[37] Westermeier F, Puebla C, Vega JL, Farias M, Escudero C, Casanello P, et al. (2009) Equilibrative nucleoside transporters in fetal endothelial dysfunction in diabetes mellitus and hyperglycaemia. Current Vascular Pharmacology 7:435-449.

[38] Farias M, Puebla C, Westermeier F, Jo MJ, Pastor-Anglada M, Casanello P, et al. (2010) Nitric oxide reduces SLC29A1 promoter activity and adenosine transport involving transcription factor complex hCHOP-C/EBPalpha in human umbilical vein endothelial cells from gestational diabetes. Cardiovascular Research 86:45-54.

[39] Westermeier F, Salomon C, Gonzalez M, Puebla C, Guzman-Gutierrez E, Cifuentes F, et al. (2011) Insulin Restores Gestational Diabetes Mellitus-Reduced Adenosine Transport Involving Differential Expression of Insulin Receptor Isoforms in Human Umbilical Vein Endothelium. Diabetes 60:1677-1687.

[40] Casanello P, Sobrevia L (2002) Intrauterine growth retardation is associated with reduced activity and expression of the cationic amino acid transport systems y+/hCAT-1 and y+/hCAT-2B and lower activity of nitric oxide synthase in human umbilical vein endothelial cells. Circulation Research 91:127-134.

[41] Escudero C, Sobrevia L (2008) A hypothesis for preeclampsia: adenosine and inducible nitric oxide synthase in human placental microvascular endothelium. Placenta 29:469-483.

[42] Casanello P, Escudero C, Sobrevia L (2007) quilibrative nucleoside (ENTs) and cationic amino acid (CATs) transporters: implications in fetal endothelial dysfunction in human pregnancy diseases. Current Vascular Pharmacology 5:69-84.

[43] Sobrevia L, Gonzalez M (2009) A role for insulin on L-arginine transport in fetal endothelial dysfunction in hyperglycaemia. Placenta 7:467-474.

[44] Alderton WK, Cooper CE, Knowles RG (2001) Nitric oxide synthases: structure, function and inhibition. Biochemical Journal 357: 593-615.

[45] Moncada S, Higgs EA (2006) Nitric oxide and the vascular endothelium. Handbook of Experimental Pharmacology 176:213-254.

[46] Ogonowski AA, Kaesemeyer WH, Jin L, Ganapathy V, Leibach FH, Caldwell RW (2000) Effects of NO donors and synthase agonists on endothelial cell uptake of L-Arg and superoxide production. American Journal of Physiology, Cell Physiology 278:C136-C143.

[47] Closs EI, Scheld JS, Sharafi M, Forstermann U (2000) Substrate supply for nitric-oxide synthase in macrophages and endothelial cells: role of cationic amino acid transporters. Molecular Pharmacology 57:68-74.

[48] De Meyer GR, Herman AG (1997) Vascular endothelial dysfunction. Progress in cardiovascular diseases 39:325-342.

[49] Deves R, Boyd CA (1998) Transporters for cationic amino acids in animal cells: discovery, structure, and function. Physiological reviews 78:487-545.

[50] Verrey F, Closs EI, Wagner CA, Palacin M, Endou H, Kanai Y (2004) CATs and HATs: the SLC7 family of amino acid transporters. European journal of physiology 447:532-542.

[51] Mann GE, Yudilevich DL, Sobrevia L (2003) Regulation of amino acid and glucose transporters in endothelial and smooth muscle cells. Physiological reviews 83:183-252.

[52] Flores C, Rojas S, Aguayo C, Parodi J, Mann G, Pearson JD, et al. (2003) Rapid stimulation of L-arginine transport by D-glucose involves p42/44(mapk) and nitric oxide in human umbilical vein endothelium. Circulation research 92:64-72.

[53] Vasquez G, Sanhueza F, Vasquez R, Gonzalez M, San Martin R, Casanello P, et al (2004) Role of adenosine transport in gestational diabetes-induced L-arginine transport and nitric oxide synthesis in human umbilical vein endothelium. The journal of physiology 560:111-122.

[54] Gonzalez M, Gallardo V, Rodriguez N, Salomon C, Westermeier F, Guzman-Gutierrez E, et al. (2011) Insulin-stimulated L-arginine transport requires SLC7A1 gene expression and is associated with human umbilical vein relaxation. Journal of cellular physiology 226:2916-2924.

[55] Cooke JP, Dzau VJ (1997) Nitric oxide synthase: role in the genesis of vascular disease. Annual review of medicine 48:489-509.

[56] Shimokawa H (1999) Primary endothelial dysfunction: atherosclerosis. Journal of molecular and cellular cardiology 31:23-37.

[57] Cai H, Harrison DG (2000) Endothelial dysfunction in cardiovascular diseases: the role of oxidant stress. Circulation research 87:840-844.

[58] Davignon J, Ganz P (2004) Role of endothelial dysfunction in atherosclerosis. Circulation 109:27-32.

[59] Walsh JH, Yong G, Cheetham C, Watts GF, O'Driscoll GJ, Taylor RR, et al. (2003) Effects of exercise training on conduit and resistance vessel function in treated and untreated hypercholesterolaemic subjects. European heart journal 24:1681-1689.

[60] Ingram DG, Newcomer SC, Price EM, Eklund KE, McAllister RM, Laughlin MH (2007) Chronic nitric oxide synthase inhibition blunts endothelium-dependent function of conduit coronary arteries, not arterioles. American journal of physiology - Heart and circulatory physiology 292:H2798-H2808.

[61] Tanner FC, Boulanger CM, Luscher TF (1993) Endothelium-derived nitric oxide, endothelin, and platelet vessel wall interaction: alterations in hypercholesterolemia and atherosclerosis. Seminars In Thrombosis And Hemostasis 19:167-175.

[62] Mathew V, Cannan CR, Miller VM, Barber DA, Hasdai D, Schwartz RS, et al. (1997) Enhanced endothelin-mediated coronary vasoconstriction and attenuated basal nitric oxide activity in experimental hypercholesterolemia. Circulation 96:1930-1936.

[63] Casino PR, Kilcoyne CM, Quyyumi AA, Hoeg JM, Panza JA (1993) The role of nitric oxide in endothelium-dependent vasodilation of hypercholesterolemic patients. Circulation 88:2541-2547.

[64] Wennmalm A (1994) Nitric oxide (NO) in the cardiovascular system: role in atherosclerosis and hypercholesterolemia. Blood Pressure 3:279-282.

[65] Laroia ST, Ganti AK, Laroia AT, Tendulkar KK (2003) Endothelium and the lipid metabolism: the current understanding. International Journal of Cardiology 88:1-9.

[66] Napoli C, Ignarro LJ (2009) Nitric oxide and pathogenic mechanisms involved in the development of vascular diseases. Archives of Pharmacal Research 32:1103-1108.

[67] Searle A, Gomez-Rosso L, Merono T, Salomon C, Duran-Sandoval D, Giunta G, et al. (2011) High LDL levels are associated with increased lipoprotein-associated phospholipase A(2) activity on nitric oxide synthesis and reactive oxygen species formation in human endothelial cells. Clinical Biochemistry 44:171-177.

[68] Verbeuren TJ, Jordaens FH, Zonnekeyn LL, Van Hove CE, Coene MC, Herman AG (1986) Effect of hypercholesterolemia on vascular reactivity in the rabbit. I. Endothelium-dependent and endothelium-independent contractions and relaxations in isolated arteries of control and hypercholesterolemic rabbits. Circulation research 58:552-564.

[69] Galle J, Busse R, Bassenge E (1991) Hypercholesterolemia and atherosclerosis change vascular reactivity in rabbits by different mechanisms. Arteriosclerosis and thrombosis : a journal of vascular biology / American Heart Association 11:1712-1718.

[70] Gilligan DM, Guetta V, Panza JA, Garcia CE, Quyyumi AA, Cannon RO (1994) Selective loss of microvascular endothelial function in human hypercholesterolemia. Circulation 90:35-41.

[71] Stapleton PA, Goodwill AG, James ME, Frisbee JC (2007) Altered mechanisms of endothelium-dependent dilation in skeletal muscle arterioles with genetic hypercholesterolemia. American Journal of Physiology,Regulatory, Integrative and Comparative Physiology 293:R1110-R1119.

[72] Stapleton PA, Goodwill AG, James ME, Brock RW, Frisbee JC (2010) Hypercholesterolemia and microvascular dysfunction: interventional strategies. Journal of Inflammation 7:54.

[73] Forstermann U, Mugge A, Alheid U, Haverich A, Frolich JC (1988) Selective attenuation of endothelium-mediated vasodilation in atherosclerotic human coronary arteries. Circulation research 62:185-190.

[74] Posch K, Simecek S, Wascher TC, Jurgens G, Baumgartner-Parzer S, Kostner GM, et al. (1999) Glycated low-density lipoprotein attenuates shear stress-induced nitric oxide synthesis by inhibition of shear stress-activated L-arginine uptake in endothelial cells. Diabetes 48:1331-1337.

[75] Jimenez A, Arriero MM, Lopez-Blaya A, Gonzalez-Fernandez F, Garcia R, Fortes J, et al. (2001) Regulation of endothelial nitric oxide synthase expression in the vascular wall and in mononuclear cells from hypercholesterolemic rabbits. Circulation 104:1822-1830.

[76] Vidal F, Colome C, Martinez-Gonzalez J, Badimon L (1998) Atherogenic concentrations of native low-density lipoproteins down-regulate nitric-oxide-synthase mRNA and protein levels in endothelial cells. European journal of biochemistry 252:378-384.

[77] Blair A, Shaul PW, Yuhanna IS, Conrad PA, Smart EJ (1999) Oxidized low density lipoprotein displaces endothelial nitric-oxide synthase (eNOS) from plasmalemmal caveolae and impairs eNOS activation. The Journal of Biological Chemistry 274:32512-32519.

[78] Feron O, Dessy C, Moniotte S, Desager JP, Balligand JL (1999) Hypercholesterolemia decreases nitric oxide production by promoting the interaction of caveolin and endothelial nitric oxide synthase. The Journal of clinical investigation 103:897-905.

[79] Everson WV, Smart EJ (2001) Influence of caveolin, cholesterol, and lipoproteins on nitric oxide synthase: implications for vascular disease. Trends in Cardiovascular Medicine 11:246-250.

[80] Feron O, Dessy C, Desager JP, Balligand JL (2001) Hydroxy-methylglutaryl-coenzyme A reductase inhibition promotes endothelial nitric oxide synthase activation through a decrease in caveolin abundance. Circulation 103:113-118.

[81] Shaul PW (2002) Regulation of endothelial nitric oxide synthase: location, location, location. Annual Review of Physiology 64:749-774.

[82] Zhu Y, Liao HL, Niu XL, Yuan Y, Lin T, Verna L, et al. (2003) Low density lipoprotein induces eNOS translocation to membrane caveolae: the role of RhoA activation and stress fiber formation. Biochimica et Biophysica Acta 1635:117-126.

[83] Michel T, Vanhoutte PM (2010) Cellular signaling and NO production. Pflügers archiv - European journal of physiology 459:807-816.

[84] Garcia-Cardena G, Fan R, Stern DF, Liu J, Sessa WC (1996) Endothelial nitric oxide synthase is regulated by tyrosine phosphorylation and interacts with caveolin-1. The Journal of Biological Chemistry 271:27237-27240.

[85] Shaul PW, Smart EJ, Robinson LJ, German Z, Yuhanna IS, Ying Y, et al. (1996) Acylation targets emdothelial nitric-oxide synthase to plasmalemmal caveolae. The Journal of Biological Chemistry 271:6518-6522.

[86] Liu J, Garcia-Cardena G, Sessa WC (1996) Palmitoylation of endothelial nitric oxide synthase is necessary for optimal stimulated release of nitric oxide: implications for caveolae localization. Biochemistry 35:13277-13281.

[87] Michel JB, Feron O, Sacks D, Michel T (1997) Reciprocal regulation of endothelial nitric-oxide synthase by Ca2+-calmodulin and caveolin. The Journal of Biological Chemistry 272:15583-15586.

[88] Bist A, Fielding PE, Fielding CJ (1997) Two sterol regulatory element-like sequences mediate up-regulation of caveolin gene transcription in response to low density lipoprotein free cholesterol. Proceedings of the National Academy of Sciences U S A 94:10693-10698.

[89] Fielding CJ, Bist A, Fielding PE (1997) Caveolin mRNA levels are up-regulated by free cholesterol and down-regulated by oxysterols in fibroblast monolayers. Proceedings of the National Academy of Sciences U S A 94:3753-3758.

[90] Hailstones D, Sleer LS, Parton RG, Stanley KK (1998) Regulation of caveolin and caveolae by cholesterol in MDCK cells. The Journal of Lipid Research 39:369-379.

[91] Boger RH, Bode-Boger SM, Szuba A, Tsao PS, Chan JR, Tangphao O, et al. (1998) Asymmetric dimethylarginine (ADMA): a novel risk factor for endothelial dysfunction: its role in hypercholesterolemia. Circulation 98:1842-1847.

[92] Boger RH, Bode-Boger SM (2000) Asymmetric dimethylarginine, derangements of the endothelial nitric oxide synthase pathway, and cardiovascular diseases. Seminars In Thrombosis And Hemostasis 26:539-545.

[93] White V, Gonzalez E, Capobianco E, Pustovrh C, Sonez C, Romanini MC, et al. (2004) Modulatory effect of leptin on nitric oxide production and lipid metabolism in term placental tissues from control and streptozotocin-induced diabetic rats. Reproduction, Fertility and Development 16:363-372.

[94] Vladimirova-Kitova L, Deneva T, Angelova E, Nikolov F, Marinov B, Mateva N (2008) Relationship of asymmetric dimethylarginine with flow-mediated dilatation in

subjects with newly detected severe hypercholesterolemia. Clinical Physiology and Functional Imaging 28:417-425.

[95] Leiper J, Nandi M (2011) The therapeutic potential of targeting endogenous inhibitors of nitric oxide synthesis. Nature Reviews Drug Discovery 10:277-291.

[96] Boger RH, Sydow K, Borlak J, Thum T, Lenzen H, Schubert B, et al. (2000) LDL cholesterol upregulates synthesis of asymmetrical dimethylarginine in human endothelial cells: involvement of S-adenosylmethionine-dependent methyltransferases. Circulation research 87:99-105.

[97] Ito A, Tsao PS, Adimoolam S, Kimoto M, Ogawa T, Cooke JP (1999) Novel mechanism for endothelial dysfunction: dysregulation of dimethylarginine dimethylaminohydrolase. Circulation 99:3092-3095.

[98] Kawashima S, Yokoyama M (2004) Dysfunction of endothelial nitric oxide synthase and atherosclerosis. Arteriosclerosis, Thrombosis, and Vascular Biology 24:998-1005.

[99] Ozaki M, Kawashima S, Yamashita T, Hirase T, Namiki M, Inoue N, et al. (2002) Overexpression of endothelial nitric oxide synthase accelerates atherosclerotic lesion formation in apoE-deficient mice. The Journal of clinical investigation 110:331-340.

[100] Tang FT, Qian ZY, Liu PQ, Zheng SG, He SY, Bao LP, et al. (2006) Crocetin improves endothelium-dependent relaxation of thoracic aorta in hypercholesterolemic rabbit by increasing eNOS activity. Biochemical Pharmacology 72:558-565.

[101] Stroes E, Kastelein J, Cosentino F, Erkelens W, Wever R, Koomans H, et al. (1997) Tetrahydrobiopterin restores endothelial function in hypercholesterolemia. The Journal of clinical investigation 99:41-46.

[102] Tiefenbacher CP, Bleeke T, Vahl C, Amann K, Vogt A, Kubler W (2000) Endothelial dysfunction of coronary resistance arteries is improved by tetrahydrobiopterin in atherosclerosis. Circulation 102:2172-2179.

[103] Tachibana D, Fukumasu H, Shintaku H, Fukumasu Y, Yamamasu S, Ishiko O, et al. (2002) Decreased plasma tetrahydrobiopterin in pregnant women is caused by impaired 6-pyruvoyl tetrahydropterin synthase activity. International Journal of Molecular Medicine 9:49-52.

[104] Iwanaga N, Yamamasu S, Tachibana D, Nishio J, Nakai Y, Shintaku H, et al. (2004) Activity of synthetic enzymes of tetrahydrobiopterin in the human placenta. International Journal of Molecular Medicine 13:117-120.

[105] Dulak J, Polus M, Guevara I, Hartwich J, Wybranska I, Krzesz R, et al. (1999) Oxidized low density lipoprotein inhibits inducible nitric oxide synthase, GTP cyclohydrolase I and transforming growth factor beta gene expression in rat macrophages. Journal of Physiology and Pharmacology 50:429-441.

[106] Dulak J, Polus M, Guevara I, Polus A, Hartwich J, Dembinska-Kiec A (1997) Regulation of inducible nitric oxide synthase (iNOS) and GTP cyclohydrolase I (GTP-CH I)

gene expression by ox-LDL in rat vascular smooth muscle cells. Journal of Physiology and Pharmacology 48:689-697.

[107] Gonzalez M, Flores C, Pearson JD, Casanello P, Sobrevia L (2004) Cell signalling-mediating insulin increase of mRNA expression for cationic amino acid transporters-1 and -2 and membrane hyperpolarization in human umbilical vein endothelial cells. Pflügers archiv - European journal of physiology 448:383-394.

[108] González M, Puebla C, Guzmán-Gutierrez E, Cifuentes F, Nien J, Abarzua F, et al. (2011) Maternal and fetal metabolic dysfunction in pregnancy diseases associated with vascular oxidative and nitrosative stress. Book: the molecular basis for the link between maternal health and the origin of the fetal congenital abnormalities 8:98-115.

[109] Jay MT, Chirico S, Siow RC, Bruckdorfer KR, Jacobs M, Leake DS, et al. (1997) Modulation of vascular tone by low density lipoproteins: effects on L-arginine transport and nitric oxide synthesis. Experimental Physiology 82:349-360.

[110] Nuszkowski A, Grabner R, Marsche G, Unbehaun A, Malle E, Heller R (2001) Hypochlorite-modified low density lipoprotein inhibits nitric oxide synthesis in endothelial cells via an intracellular dislocalization of endothelial nitric-oxide synthase. The Journal of Biological Chemistry 276:14212-14221.

[111] Kikuta K, Sawamura T, Miwa S, Hashimoto N, Masaki T (1998) High-affinity arginine transport of bovine aortic endothelial cells is impaired by lysophosphatidylcholine. Circulation research 83:1088-1096.

[112] Vergnani L, Hatrik S, Ricci F, Passaro A, Manzoli N, Zuliani G, et al. (2000) Effect of native and oxidized low-density lipoprotein on endothelial nitric oxide and superoxide production : key role of L-arginine availability. Circulation 101:1261-1266.

[113] Zhang WZ, Venardos K, Finch S, Kaye DM (2008) Detrimental effect of oxidized LDL on endothelial arginine metabolism and transportation. The International Journal of Biochemistry and Cell Biology 40:920-928.

[114] Ryoo S, Bhunia A, Chang F, Shoukas A, Berkowitz DE, Romer LH (2011) OxLDL-dependent activation of arginase II is dependent on the LOX-1 receptor and downstream RhoA signaling. Atherosclerosis 214:279-287.

[115] Ryoo S, Gupta G, Benjo A, Lim HK, Camara A, Sikka G, et al. (2008) Endothelial arginase II: a novel target for the treatment of atherosclerosis. Circulation research 102:923-932.

[116] Erdely A, Kepka-Lenhart D, Salmen-Muniz R, Chapman R, Hulderman T, Kashon M, et al. (2010) Arginase activities and global arginine bioavailability in wild-type and ApoE-deficient mice: responses to high fat and high cholesterol diets. PLoS One 5:e15253.

[117] Holowatz LA, Santhanam L, Webb A, Berkowitz DE, Kenney WL (2011) Oral atorvastatin therapy restores cutaneous microvascular function by decreasing arginase activity in hypercholesterolaemic humans. The journal of physiology 589:2093-2103.

[118] Metzger BE, Coustan DR (1998) Summary and recommendations of the Fourth International Workshop-Conference on Gestational Diabetes Mellitus. The Organizing Committee. Diabetes Care 21:S161-S167.

[119] Metzger BE, Buchanan TA, Coustan DR, de Leiva A, Dunger DB, Hadden DR, et al. (2007) Summary and recommendations of the Fifth International Workshop-Conference on Gestational Diabetes Mellitus. Diabetes Care 30:S251-S260.

[120] American Diabetes Association (2011) Diagnosis and classification of diabetes mellitus. Diabetes Care 34:S62-S69.

[121] Nold JL, Georgieff MK (2004) Infants of diabetic mothers. Pediatric Clinics of North America 51:619-637.

[122] Greene MF, Solomon CG (2005) Gestational diabetes mellitus -- time to treat. The New England Journal of Medicine 352:2544-2546.

[123] Desoye G, Hauguel-de Mouzon S (2007) The human placenta in gestational diabetes mellitus. The insulin and cytokine network. Diabetes Care 33:S120-S126.

[124] Belmar J C, Salinas C P, Becker V J, Abarzúa C F, Olmos C P, González B P, et al. (2004) Incidencia de diabetes gestacional segun distintos metodos diagnosticos y sus implicancias clinicas. Revista Chilena de Obstetricia y Ginecología 69:2-7.

[125] Huidobro A, Fulford A, Carrasco E (2004) Incidence of gestational diabetes and relationship to obesity in Chilean pregnant women. Revista Medica de Chile 132:931-938.

[126] Ferrara A, Kahn HS, Quesenberry CP, Riley C, Hedderson MM (2004) An increase in the incidence of gestational diabetes mellitus: Northern California, 1991-2000. Obstetrics and Gynecology 103:526-533.

[127] Dabelea D, Snell-Bergeon JK, Hartsfield CL, Bischoff KJ, Hamman RF, McDuffie RS (2005) Increasing prevalence of gestational diabetes mellitus (GDM) over time and by birth cohort: Kaiser Permanente of Colorado GDM Screening Program. Diabetes Care 28:579-584.

[128] Robitaille J, Grant AM (2008) The genetics of gestational diabetes mellitus: evidence for relationship with type 2 diabetes mellitus. Genetics in Medicine 10:240-250.

[129] Omar HA, Ramirez R, Arsich J, Tracy T, Glover D, Gibson M (1998) Reduction of the Human Placental Vascular Relaxation to Progesterone by Gestational Diabetes. Journal of Maternal-Fetal Investigation 8:27-30.

[130] De Vriese AS, Verbeuren TJ, Van de Voorde J, Lameire NH, Vanhoutte PM (2000) Endothelial dysfunction in diabetes. British Journal of Pharmacology 130:963-974.

[131] Tchirikov M, Rybakowski C, Huneke B, Schoder V, Schroder HJ (2002) Umbilical vein blood volume flow rate and umbilical artery pulsatility as 'venous-arterial index' in the prediction of neonatal compromise. Ultrasound Obstetrics and Gynecology 20:580-585.

[132] Biri A, Onan A, Devrim E, Babacan F, Kavutcu M, Durak I (2006) Oxidant status in maternal and cord plasma and placental tissue in gestational diabetes. Placenta 27:327-332.

[133] Guzman-Gutierrez E, Westermeier F, Salomon C, Gonzalez M, Pardo F, Leiva A, et al. (2012) Insulin-Increased L-Arginine Transport Requires A(2A) Adenosine Receptors Activation in Human Umbilical Vein Endothelium. PLoS One 7:e41705.

[134] Salomon C, Westermeier F, Puebla C, Arroyo P, Guzman-Gutierrez E, Pardo F, et al. (2012) Gestational diabetes reduces adenosine transport in human placental microvascular endothelium, an effect reversed by insulin. PLoS One 7:e40578.

[135] von Mandach U, Lauth D, Huch R (2003) Maternal and fetal nitric oxide production in normal and abnormal pregnancy. Journal of Maternal-Fetal and Neonatal Medicine 13:22-27.

[136] Farias M, San Martin R, Puebla C, Pearson JD, Casado JF, Pastor-Anglada M, et al. (2006) Nitric oxide reduces adenosine transporter ENT1 gene (SLC29A1) promoter activity in human fetal endothelium from gestational diabetes. Journal of cellular physiology 208:451-460.

[137] National Cholesterol Education Program (NCEP) Expert Panel on Detection, Evaluation, and Treatment of High Blood Cholesterol in Adults (Adult Treatment Panel III) (2002) Third Report of the National Cholesterol Education Program (NCEP) Expert Panel on Detection, Evaluation, and Treatment of High Blood Cholesterol in Adults (Adult Treatment Panel III) final report. Circulation 106:3143-3421.

[138] Roger VL, Go AS, Lloyd-Jones DM, Adams RJ, Berry JD, Brown TM, et al. (2011) Heart Disease and Stroke Statistics--2011 Update: A Report From the American Heart Association. Circulation 123:e18-e209.

[139] Arsenault BJ, Boekholdt SM, Kastelein JJ (2011) Lipid parameters for measuring risk of cardiovascular disease. Nature Reviews Cardiology 8:197-206.

[140] Boney CM, Verma A, Tucker R, Vohr BR (2005) Metabolic syndrome in childhood: association with birth weight, maternal obesity, and gestational diabetes mellitus. Pediatrics 115:e290-e296.

[141] Clausen TD, Mathiesen ER, Hansen T, Pedersen O, Jensen DM, Lauenborg J, et al. (2009) Overweight and the metabolic syndrome in adult offspring of women with diet-treated gestational diabetes mellitus or type 1 diabetes. The Journal of Clinical Endocrinology and Metabolism 94:2464-2470.

[142] Moore TR (2010) Fetal exposure to gestational diabetes contributes to subsequent adult metabolic syndrome. American Journal of Obstetrics and Gynecology 202:643-649.

[143] Isomaa B, Almgren P, Tuomi T, Forsen B, Lahti K, Nissen M, et al. (2001) Cardiovascular morbidity and mortality associated with the metabolic syndrome. Diabetes Care 24:683-689.

[144] Egeland GM, Meltzer SJ. (2010) Following in mother's footsteps? Mother-daughter risks for insulin resistance and cardiovascular disease 15 years after gestational diabetes. Diabetic Medicine 27:257-265.

[145] Pirkola J, Vaarasmaki M, Ala-Korpela M, Bloigu A, Canoy D, Hartikainen AL, et al. (2010) Low-grade, systemic inflammation in adolescents: association with early-life factors, gender, and lifestyle. American Journal of Epidemiology 171:72-82.

[146] Mottillo S, Filion KB, Genest J, Joseph L, Pilote L, Poirier P, et al. (2010) The metabolic syndrome and cardiovascular risk a systematic review and meta-analysis. Journal of the American College of Cardiology 56:1113-1132.

[147] Sanchez-Vera I, Bonet B, Viana M, Quintanar A, Martin MD, Blanco P, et al. (2007) Changes in plasma lipids and increased low-density lipoprotein susceptibility to oxidation in pregnancies complicated by gestational diabetes: consequences of obesity. Metabolism 56:1527-1533.

[148] Zawiejska A, Wender-Ozegowska E, Brazert J, Sodowski K (2008) Components of metabolic syndrome and their impact on fetal growth in women with gestational diabetes mellitus. Journal of Physiology and Pharmacology 59:5-18.

[149] Reece E. (2010) The fetal and maternal consequences of gestational diabetes mellitus. Journal of Maternal-Fetal and Neonatal Medicine 23:199-203.

[150] Radaelli T, Lepercq J, Varastehpour A, Basu S, Catalano PM, Hauguel-De Mouzon S (2009) Differential regulation of genes for fetoplacental lipid pathways in pregnancy with gestational and type 1 diabetes mellitus. American Journal of Obstetrics and Gynecology 201:209 e201-209 e210.

[151] Scholler M, Wadsack C, Lang I, Etschmaier K, Schweinzer C, Marsche G, et al. (2012) Phospholipid transfer protein in the placental endothelium is affected by gestational diabetes mellitus. The Journal of Clinical Endocrinology and Metabolism 97:437-445.

[152] Marceau G, Volle DH, Gallot D, Mangelsdorf DJ, Sapin V, Lobaccaro JM (2005) Placental expression of the nuclear receptors for oxysterols LXRalpha and LXRbeta during mouse and human development. The anatomical record. Part A, Discoveries in molecular, cellular, and evolutionary biology 283:175-181.

[153] Scholler M, Wadsack C, Metso J, Chirackal Manavalan AP, Sreckovic I, Schweinzer C, et al. (2012) Phospholipid Transfer Protein Is Differentially Expressed in Human

Arterial and Venous Placental Endothelial Cells and Enhances Cholesterol Efflux to Fetal HDL. The Journal of Clinical Endocrinology and Metabolism 97:2466-2474.

[154] Ferderbar S, Pereira EC, Apolinario E, Bertolami MC, Faludi A, Monte O, et al. (2007) Cholesterol oxides as biomarkers of oxidative stress in type 1 and type 2 diabetes mellitus. Diabetes/Metabolism Research and Reviews 23:35-42.

[155] Skilton MR (2008) Intrauterine risk factors for precocious atherosclerosis. Pediatrics 121:570-574.

[156] Sarikabadayi YU, Aydemir O, Kanmaz G, Aydemir C, Oguz SS, Erdeve O, et al. (2012) Umbilical artery intima-media and wall thickness in infants of diabetic mothers. Neonatology 102:157-162.

[157] Vahratian A, Misra VK, Trudeau S, Misra DP (2010) Prepregnancy body mass index and gestational age-dependent changes in lipid levels during pregnancy. Obstetrics and Gynecology 116:107-113.

[158] Knopp RH, Van Allen MI, McNeely M, Walden CE, Plovie B, Shiota K, et al. (1993) Effect of insulin-dependent diabetes on plasma lipoproteins in diabetic pregnancy. The Journal of Reproductive Medicine 38:703-710.

[159] Vanderjagt DJ, Patel RJ, El-Nafaty AU, Melah GS, Crossey MJ, Glew RH (2004) High-density lipoprotein and homocysteine levels correlate inversely in preeclamptic women in northern Nigeria. Acta Obstetricia et Gynecologica Scandinavica 83:536-542.

[160] Ywaskewycz L BG, Castillo MS,López D, Pedrozo W (2010) Perfil lipídico por trimestre de gestación en una poblacion de mujeres adultas. Revista Chilena de Obstetricia y Ginecología 75:227-233.

[161] Sattar N, Greer IA, Louden J, Lindsay G, McConnell M, Shepherd J, et al. (1997) Lipoprotein subfraction changes in normal pregnancy: threshold effect of plasma triglyceride on appearance of small, dense low density lipoprotein. The Journal of Clinical Endocrinology and Metabolism 82:2483-2491.

[162] Martin U, Davies C, Hayavi S, Hartland A, Dunne F (1999) Is normal pregnancy atherogenic? Clinical Science 96:421-425.

[163] Koukkou E, Watts GF, Mazurkiewicz J, Lowy C (1994) Ethnic differences in lipid and lipoprotein metabolism in pregnant women of African and Caucasian origin. Journal of Clinical Pathology 47:1105-1107.

[164] Mazurkiewicz JC, Watts GF, Warburton FG, Slavin BM, Lowy C, Koukkou E (1994) Serum lipids, lipoproteins and apolipoproteins in pregnant non-diabetic patients. Journal of Clinical Pathology 47:728-731.

[165] Liguori A, D'Armiento FP, Palagiano A, Balestrieri ML, Williams-Ignarro S, de Nigris F, et al. (2007) Effect of gestational hypercholesterolaemia on omental vasoreactivity,

placental enzyme activity and transplacental passage of normal and oxidised fatty acids. BJOG: An International Journal of Obstetrics and Gynaecology 114:1547-1556.

[166] Magnussen EB, Vatten LJ, Smith GD, Romundstad PR (2009) Hypertensive disorders in pregnancy and subsequently measured cardiovascular risk factors. Obstetrics and Gynecology 114:961-970.

[167] Bon C, Raudrant D, Golfier F, Poloce F, Champion F, Pichot J, et al. (2007) [Feto-maternal metabolism in human normal pregnancies: study of 73 cases]. Annales de biologie clinique 65:609-619.

[168] Schaefer-Graf UM, Graf K, Kulbacka I, Kjos SL, Dudenhausen J, Vetter K, et al. (2008) Maternal lipids as strong determinants of fetal environment and growth in pregnancies with gestational diabetes mellitus. Diabetes Care 31:1858-1863.

[169] Ordovas JM, Pocovi M, Grande F (1984) Plasma lipids and cholesterol esterification rate during pregnancy. Obstetrics and Gynecology 63:20-25.

[170] Belo L, Caslake M, Gaffney D, Santos-Silva A, Pereira-Leite L, Quintanilha A, et al. (2002) Changes in LDL size and HDL concentration in normal and preeclamptic pregnancies. Atherosclerosis 162:425-432.

[171] Saarelainen H, Laitinen T, Raitakari OT, Juonala M, Heiskanen N, Lyyra-Laitinen T, et al. (2006) Pregnancy-related hyperlipidemia and endothelial function in healthy women. Circulation Journal 70:768-772.

[172] Ogura K, Miyatake T, Fukui O, Nakamura T, Kameda T, Yoshino G (2002) Low-density lipoprotein particle diameter in normal pregnancy and preeclampsia. Journal of Atherosclerosis and Thrombosis 9:42-47.

[173] Ouyang Y, Chen H, Chen H (2007) Reduced plasma adiponectin and elevated leptin in pre-eclampsia. International Journal of Gynecology and Obstetrics 98:110-114.

[174] Iftikhar U, Iqbal A, Shakoor S (2010) Relationship between leptin and lipids during pre-eclampsia. Journal of the Pakistan Medical Association 60:432-435.

[175] Mshelia DS, Kullima A, Gali RM, Kawuwa MB, Mamza YP, Habu SA, et al. (2010) The use of plasma lipid and lipoprotein ratios in interpreting the hyperlipidaemia of pregnancy. Journal of obstetrics and gynaecology 30:804-808.

[176] Grissa O, Ategbo JM, Yessoufou A, Tabka Z, Miled A, Jerbi M, et al. (2007) Antioxidant status and circulating lipids are altered in human gestational diabetes and macrosomia. Translational Research 150:164-171.

[177] Rossmanith WG, Hoffmeister U, Wolfahrt S, Kleine B, McLean M, Jacobs RA, et al. (1999) Expression and functional analysis of endothelial nitric oxide synthase (eNOS) in human placenta. Molecular Human Reproduction 5:487-494.

[178] Di Iulio JL, Gude NM, King RG, Li CG, Rand MJ, Brennecke SP (1999)Human placental nitric oxide synthase activity is not altered in diabetes. Clinical Science 97:123-128.

[179] Thornburg KL, O'Tierney PF, Louey S (2010) Review: The placenta is a programming agent for cardiovascular disease. Placenta 31:S54-S59.

[180] Lee MY, Cai Y, Wang Y, Liao SY, Liu Y, Zhang Y, et al. (2012) Differential genomic changes caused by cholesterol- and PUFA-rich diets in regenerated porcine coronary endothelial cells. Physiological Genomics 44:551-561.

[181] Chan E, Chan JY, Wu JH, Wan CW, Leung GP, Lee SM, et al. (2012) Serum nitric oxide synthase activity is a novel predictor of impaired vasorelaxation in rats. Clinical and Experimental Pharmacology and Physiology 39:894-896.

[182] Kim OY, Lee SM, Chung JH, Do HJ, Moon J, Shin MJ (2012) Arginase I and the very low-density lipoprotein receptor are associated with phenotypic biomarkers for obesity. Nutrition 28:635-639.

[183] Hollingsworth DR, Grundy SM (1982) Pregnancy-associated hypertriglyceridemia in normal and diabetic women. Differences in insulin-dependent, non-insulin-dependent, and gestational diabetes. Diabetes 31:1092-1097.

[184] Tarim E, Yigit F, Kilicdag E, Bagis T, Demircan S, Simsek E, et al. (2006) Early onset of subclinical atherosclerosis in women with gestational diabetes mellitus. Ultrasound Obstetrics and Gynecology 27:177-182.

[185] Koukkou E, Watts GF, Lowy C (1996) Serum lipid, lipoprotein and apolipoprotein changes in gestational diabetes mellitus: a cross-sectional and prospective study. Journal of Clinical Pathology 49:634-637.

[186] Knopp RH, LaRosa JC, Burkman RT (1993) Contraception and dyslipidemia. American Journal of Obstetrics and Gynecology 168:1994-2005.

[187] Rizzo M, Berneis K, Altinova AE, Toruner FB, Akturk M, Ayvaz G, et al. (2008) Atherogenic lipoprotein phenotype and LDL size and subclasses in women with gestational diabetes. Diabetic Medicine 25:1406-1411.

Chapter 7

The Role of Placenta in the Fetal Programming Associated to Gestational Diabetes

Carlos Escudero, Marcelo González, Jesenia Acurio, Francisco Valenzuela and Luis Sobrevia

Additional information is available at the end of the chapter

http://dx.doi.org/10.5772/55384

1. Introduction

Gestational diabetes mellitus (GDM) is a human pregnancy disease characterized by elevation of glucose levels (i.e., hyperglycemia) responsible for a several adverse perinatal outcomes included macrosomia, fetal hypoglycemia, requirement of neonatal intensive care and neonatal mortality, among others. Estimation of the epidemiological impact of GDM has indicated that at least 1 out of 10 pregnant woman is being affected by GDM worldwide. In addition, GDM causes not only short-term complication in both mother and fetus, but also is associated with elevated risk for long-term complication such as cardiovascular disease, obesity and diabetes. Even though it is not feasible to exclude the genetic component in the elevated risk for metabolic/cardiovascular disease later in life, the general agreement is that hyperglycemia generates an adaptive response in the fetus addressing to control the glucose level, characterized by hyperinsulinemia. Part of this adaptive response, might also include the elevation in the placental consumption of glucose and enhancement of the feto-placental blood flow, especially in fetus large-for-gestational age (LGA). On the other hand, due to lack of innervation in the placenta, the vascular tone is controlled by the regulation of the synthesis and release of vasoactive substances from the endothelium like vasoactive molecules, nitric oxide, adenosine, prostaglandin, among others. Interestingly, vasoactive molecules may also regulate endothelial proliferation and migration, suggesting that they also affect the vessel formation (i.e., angiogenesis). In this regard, several studies have shown that placenta from GDM is characterized by hypervascularization and elevation in the pro-angiogenic signals including the secretion and activity of the vascular endothelial growth factor (VEGF). In addition, hyperglycemia also generates a status of oxidative stress, where free radicals derived from oxygen (ROS) induces changes in the endothelial cell membranes producing an elevation in the cell permeability. Therefore, it is feasible that the adaptive response -useful for surviving in a hostile medium (i.e, hyperglycemia) - may be imprinting in the fetus and once he/she is exposed to other different conditions after delivery, this response might constitute a risk factor for developing metabolic diseases. In this chapter, we will review the available literature focus on the role of feto-placental endothelial dysfunction as the possible main factor in the generation of short-term complication during GDM and speculate how it may program the response of the sibling exposed to GDM.

2. Gestational diabetes: Definition and epidemiology

Pregnancy is a physiological state where occurs a series of complex anatomical and functional adaptation in the mother to facilitate the development of fetus. For instance, during the normal pregnancy a "physiological" insulin resistance is necessary to provide glucose to the growing fetus [1]. However, this normal adaptation is no longer occurring in some conditions and generates a clearly pathological state of insulin resistance, which is called Gestational Diabetes Mellitus (GDM). Therefore, GDM has been defined as any degree of glucose intolerance with onset or first recognition during pregnancy [2]. Specifically, the World Health Organization (WHO) has stated that GDM encompasses impaired glucose tolerance and diabetes identified as fasting glucose level ≥ 7 mmol/L or ≥ 126 mg/dL; or 2 hours plasma glucose after oral glucose (75 g) tolerance test (OGTT) ≥ 7.8 mmol/L or ≥ 140 mg/dL [3]. Despite this recommendation, it has been worldwide accepted recently a new diagnosis criteria, which it has been given by the Diabetes in Pregnancy Study Group (IADPSG) based on the OGTT (fasting glucose ≥ 5.1 mmol/L or ≥ 92 mg/dl, or a one hour result of ≥ 10.0 mmol/L or ≥ 180 mg/dl, or a two hours result of ≥ 8.5 mmol/L or ≥ 153 mg/dL), which is still controversial based on the analysis of the risk for perinatal adverse outcomes [2]. This discrepancy has been extensively discussed in the literature but the general agreement is that adverse perinatal outcomes occur in lesser degrees of hyperglycemia than the recommended as diagnostic criteria by the WHO [4].

Prevalence of diabetes for all ages is increasing worldwide, including women in fertile age. Therefore, it is not surprising that diabetes diagnosis before or during gestation has been defined as a public health problem [5]. Epidemiologically speaking, it has been estimated that near to 90% of the diagnosis of diabetes in pregnancy is actually GDM [5]. More precisely, GDM affects from 1.4% to 25.5% of pregnancies, however, its incidence will depend on the population, which it has been tested and the diagnostic criteria used [6,7]. Thus, taken into account the origin of the population, it has been described that women from Asian, African American, and Hispanic background exhibit twice the risk for being diagnosed of GDM compared to those of non-Hispanic White origin, a phenomenon observed also in women in the lowest socio-economical quartiles compared to women in the highest quartiles [8,9].

The underling mechanisms responsible for GDM are under investigation; however, likewise to other causes of type 2 diabetes, GDM is characterized by a dysfunction in the pancreatic β cell, which does not produce enough insulin to meet the increased requirements of late pregnancy. Mechanistic studies reveal at least three possibilities: 1) The presence of anti-islet cell antibodies (<10% cases); 2) Genetic variants of monogenic forms of diabetes (1-5% cases), and 3) Presence of obesity and chronic insulin resistance (>80% cases) [10]. In addition, it has been described that the large majority of the insulin secretory defects present in the third trimester of gestation, are actually manifesting before and soon after pregnancy [10,11]. In this way, considering that a) obesity, is a condition of insulin resistance and a common risk factor to GDM, and b) insulin secretion during pregnancy increases according to gestational age in women with and without GDM [10]; it has been reinforced the concept that chronic deficiency rather than gestational-acquired deficiency of insulin secretion is the underling cause for GDM. Consequently, these evidences have broken the traditional vision of GDM pathogenesis, where the imbalance in glucose level at the third trimester of gestation has been consider exclusively as a defect in the "physiological" insulin resistance present in pregnant women.

With regard to insulin, it is well known that it reduces the elevated level of blood glucose; however, insulin is also regulating the metabolism of amino acids and lipids. Indeed, selective damage of β-cell in animal models generates a severe lipid defects that induce animal death [12,13]. This idea reinforces the general agreement of hyperglycemia is not the unique feature that may be taken into account during GDM management. In addition, it has been reported that in general, hyperglycemia is resolved after birth; however, there are epidemiological evidences showing that GDM constitutes a risk factor for development of diabetes mellitus type 2 (DMT2), as well as it constitutes a risk factor for hypertension in both mother and offspring. Thus, it has been estimated that about 10% of women with GDM have diabetes mellitus soon after delivery; whereas the rest will develop diabetes mellitus at rates of 20-60% within 5-10 years after the manifestation of GDM in the absence of specific interventions to reduce their risk [10]. Therefore these evidences have suggested that metabolic defects in GDM, characterized by hyperglycemia, and fundamentally, insulin deficiency (relative in GDM) are maintained after birth being a risk factor for metabolic and cardiovascular diseases in the mother and her sibling.

3. Fetal and neonatal outcomes in GDM

Gestational diabetes is associated with multiple adverse perinatal outcomes which include in the mother, haemorrhage, hypertensive disorders, obstructed labor, infection/sepsis, and maternal mortality [14]. Thus, in the Hyperglycemia and Adverse Pregnancy Outcomes (HAPO) study [4], which included a large number of participants (23.316) in nine countries, who were divided into 7 groups according with the fasting and glucose plasma level observed during OGTT; and importantly considering a level of glycaemia lower than the WHO criteria, showed a linear relationship between glucose level (both fasting and after OGTT) with the occurrence of adverse perinatal outcomes such as birth weight and cord-blood serum C-peptide level above the 90th percentile, cesarean section, neonatal hypoglycemia, premature delivery, shoulder dystosia or birth injury, intensive neonatal care, hyperbilirubinemia, and maternal pre-eclampsia. On the other hand, at the fetal side, this study describes that the higher level of glucose, the higher risk (between 1.37 and 5.01) of elevated birth weight. Thus, considering data on the difference in the birth weight between the lowest and the highest glucose categories was about 300g. Therefore, this study suggests that maternal hyperglycemia, even in the "normal" range according with the WHO criteria, is related to clinically important perinatal disorders.

Considering this report, a recent meta-analysis [2] which included a large number of patient (44.829), containing who were included in the HAPO study and using the criteria recommended by the WHO, showed that diagnosis of diabetes was associated with high risk (RR=1.37 to 1.88) for presenting macrosomia, large for gestational age, perinatal mortality, preeclampsia and cesarean delivery. When the authors excluded the HAPO study from their meta-analysis, the relative risks for the analyzed perinatal outcomes were minimally altered. Specifically, and considering the highest risk described in this meta-analysis, women with GDM exhibited a high risk for macrosomia (RR=1.81) and large for gestational age (RR=1.73). This association between GDM and macrosomia is particularly important for our discussion, since it has been described that fetal growth defects are associated with long-term complication, including obesity and diabetes [15,16]. Nevertheless, another highlight of this meta-analysis is that reduction in the criteria for "hyperglycemia" recommended by the WHO, should be considered for the next generation.

Although discrepancies in cut off value of glucose level for diagnosis of GDM, most of the alterations observed in GDM have been related with "hyperglycemia". For instance, it has been shown that intraperitoneal injections of high glucose in early pregnancy were associated with a modest but significantly increased placental weight and fetal weight [17]. Therefore, authors suggest that increased fetal growth may be explained by a large placenta and delivery of more nutrients to be transferred to the fetus. Since macrosomia is also present in "normo-glycemic" pregnant women, it has been suggested that other factors rather than high glucose by itself may take part in the pathophysiology of maternal and fetal-neonatal complication present in GDM [18]. In this way, other clinical components in GDM, included metabolic alteration such as insulin resistance, as well as high levels of cholesterol, triglycerides, adenosine, nitric oxide, and several other factors may disrupt normal function of maternal, placental and fetal tissues. Specifically, it is well accepted that hyperglycemia in the fetus exposed to GDM, generates a compensatory elevation of insulin; which in turn, is not only affecting glucose level, but also is acting as a growth factor. In addition, insulin is also regulating the transport of other nutrients such as amino acids or other regulatory elements such as adenosine [19,20,21]. In particular, it has been described that insulin increases the L-arginine uptake in human umbilical vein endothelial cells (HUVEC), a phenomenon associated with generation of vein relaxation and increasing Sp1-activated *SLC7A1* (for human cationic amino acid transport type 1, hCAT-1) expression [22]. In addition, it has been described that insulin increases the activity of neutral amino acid through the system A [23]. On the other hand, insulin recovers the reduced adenosine transport mediated by the *E*quilibrative *N*ucleside *T*ransport type 1 (ENT-1) in HUVEC, an effect that was associated with increased relaxation of the umbilical vein [24]. Therefore, the general consensus is that the fetus's tissues (and in particular the placenta) are able to generate a compensatory response characterized by hyperinsulinemia, and aimed to revert the deleterious effect of GDM (i.e., hyperglycemia) and ultimately improve fetal survive. In this context, it has been suggested that this adaptive response (i.e., fetal programming) may not match with the extrauterine environment, in both early and later life, and it would be responsible for either neonatal complications after birth or long-term diseases [15]. In the next section, it will be reviewed some of these evidences and the mechanisms linked with fetal programming in GDM.

4. Programming and GDM

Programming is defined as "the phenomenon whereby a stimulus occurring during a critical window of development, namely the prenatal and early postnatal periods, which can cause lifelong changes in the structure and function of the body" [25]. In this regard, the concept that the intrauterine environment might affect health later life became evident with the surprising observation that low birth weight was associated with increased cardiovascular disease 40 years later [15,16,26]. Numerous epidemiological studies extended these observations to suggest a role for the intrauterine environment as a leading cause of schizophrenia, depression, cardiovascular diseases, stroke, diabetes, cancer, pulmonary hypertension, osteoporosis, polycystic ovarian syndrome, among others in adult life [27,28,29,30]. These observational relationships are supported by animal experiments, which fetal growth manipulation by changing maternal nutrition or reducing blood flow to the placenta resulted in obesity, increased blood pressure and other cardiovascular abnormalities in the offspring later life [31]. As indicated, most of this observation included newborns with restricted growth but the contrary phenomenon (i.e., macrosomia) is observed in GDM.

In addition, a clear association between maternal diseases (including GDM) and future implication in health in the offspring has been affected by several confounding variables such as genetic factors (a particular phenotype may be genetically transmitted to the offspring), paternal implication (the father genotype may affect the phenotype), gender (hormonal differences may induce a particular gender-linked phenotype), diagnosis criteria used for maternal disease (in the particular case of GDM, the level of glycaemia), retrospective evidences (most of the epidemiological analysis coming from retrospective rather than prospective studies), among others. Despite those confounding factors, most of the available data in the case of GDM supports a predominant role for intrauterine exposition to hyperglycemia as one of the underling mechanisms for future chronic disease in the offspring exposed to this disease [25]. Among the evidences that support this assumption, it has been described that children born after a diabetic pregnancy in Indian Pima women exhibited a high (6-fold) prevalence of type 2 diabetes than those who were born from a non-diabetic pregnancy. Interestingly, this high prevalence persists after a multivariable analysis, taken into account paternal diabetes, age of onset of parental diabetes in father and mother and obesity in the offspring [32]. Besides, another study showed that the risk of diabetes was significantly higher (≈ 4 fold) in siblings born after GDM than those who were born before the mother has been diagnosed with diabetes [33]. In the next section we will highlight some of those evidences.

Offspring "exposed" to GDM shows a high risk for developing obesity, impaired glucose tolerance, type 2 diabetes, malignant neoplasm and hypertension in adulthood

[34,35,36,37,38,39]. For instance, initially, it has been reported that offspring (10-16 years) "exposed" to maternal diabetes showed a higher prevalence (6-fold) of impaired glucose tolerance and body mass index than controls non-exposed [40]. Furthermore, this finding was confirmed in another study including children (1-9 years) who their mothers presented pregestational insulin-dependent diabetes (IDDM) or GDM [41]. Following to this study, prospective data from the Framingham Offspring Study [42], which included a large sample (2.527 subjects), found that offspring (26-82 years) of women with diabetes showed a high risk (≈3-fold) to impaired glucose tolerance and type 2 diabetes compared to individuals without parental diabetes. This risk was almost three times higher in children belong to diabetic mothers <50 years. Moreover, another study also confirms these findings, where offspring "exposed" to GDM exhibited ≈ 7 folds increase in the prevalence of type 2 diabetes or impaired glucose tolerance compared to offspring from non-diabetic pregnancy [39]. Interestingly, this risk was even higher than offspring of women with type 1 diabetes who presented ≈ 4 fold risk for being diabetic [39], reinforcing the idea that maternal intrauterine environment generates a particular phenotype which is not explained only by heritage. Nevertheless, Clausen et al (2009) have reported a high risk (≈ 2 fold) for developing overweight or metabolic syndrome in offspring of women with GDM or type 1 diabetes compared to offspring from non-diabetic pregnancies. It has been also reported that the higher hyperglycemia in the mother [36] or the weight for gestational age in children exposed to GDM [43], the higher risk for metabolic syndrome in the offspring in future life.

Moreover, GDM is also associated with high risk for cardiovascular diseases in the offspring. Thus, in a large cohort study, it has been reported that children exposed to GDM had higher systolic blood pressure (≈3 mm Hg) than non-exposed children [44]. Moreover, other study [38], which also included children (5-9 years) "exposed" to maternal diabetes, reported a higher level of insulin resistance (i.e., HOMA index) than control subjects. On the other hand, another recent report including more than 1.7 million singleton born in Denmark found that sibling (followed for up to 30 years) "exposed" to GDM exhibited a high risk for developing malignant neoplasm (2.2-fold) and for diseases of the circulatory system (1.3-fold) [45]. Interestingly, a significantly higher risk for those groups of diseases were also observed in children whose mother had type 1 diabetes or pre-gestational type 2 diabetes. Therefore, a hyperglycemic intrauterine environment seems to be part of the pathogenesis of chronic metabolic and cardiovascular disease in the offspring of GDM [36,37,39].

The mechanisms linked with fetal programming during GDM have been associated with hyperglycemia, through the hypothesis of fuel-mediated toxicity (Freinkel's hypothesis) [46], which indicates that fetus experiences a "tissue culture" environment, in such circumstances, where high availability of nutrients may induce a "fuel-mediated teratogenicity". In this scenario, high metabolism of glucose in the fetus may generate an excessive consumption of oxygen (i.e., relative hypoxia) and consequently, it may generate an oxidative stress condition. This last phenomenon, would affect the normal development of organs or systems that are completing its development during late gestation and/or perinatal period, such as placenta, kidney and vasculature [25]. Particularly, we will focus on the alterations observed in the placental vasculature, early in life, that may support the association between elevated risk for

http://dx.doi.org/10.5772/55384

cardiovascular disease during adulthood and GDM. In this regard, two branches of the knowledge may be discuss: 1) Anatomical and functional alterations that are involved in the deregulation of placental vascular tone control [47]; and 2) Alterations in the formation of new blood vessels (i.e., angiogenesis) [48]. Since placental circulatory system form a continuous network with the fetal circulation, it is feasible to propose that changes in the function and regulation of all these vessels early after birth may give clues of the abnormalities that will occur later in life.

5. GDM and placental anatomy/histology

The placenta- endocrine organ and an immune barrier - is the functional unit where occurs the exchange of oxygen and carbon dioxide, the absorption of nutrient and the elimination of metabolic waste. The placenta prevents the passage of macromolecules over 700 Daltons, whereas the smallest particles can cross (for instance melatonin, catecholamines and other hormones) [49,50]; therefore, this tissue exhibits a selective permeability that is known as the placental barrier. In the formation of human placenta, the maternal vessels are invaded by trophoblastic cells, which in turn are in direct contact with maternal blood. This type of structure is named hemochorial placenta [51]. Two layers coexist in this structure, the maternal and the fetal one. In the maternal side, a laminar degenerative process in the junctional zone forms the maternal layer or uterine surface, which in general are formed by maternal vessels where the endothelium has been replaced by placental cells (invasive cytothrophoblast), remnants of endometrial glands and connective tissue. Moreover, grooves is shown in this structure, which subdivide the surface of placenta in about 10-40 elevated areas similar to lobules named maternal cotyledons, which are in perfect correlation with fetal cotyledon [51]. The fetal component, cotyledon, is formed by several villous trees (1-3 villous trees per fetal cotyledon), which in fact are formed by chorionic villus. This anatomic and functional structure are formed by syncytiotrophoblasts/cytotrophoblasts, stromal core villi and fetal vascular endothelium [52].

Cytotrophoblast and differentiated syncytiotrophoblast are derived from trophoblastic cells. The syncytiotrophoblast is a multinucleated and continuous layer of epithelial cells, which is formed by the fusion of cytotrophoblasts. In the other hand, syncytiotrophoblast is covering the villous trees and it is in direct contact with maternal blood, therefore, it is the area where direct exchange of oxygen, nutrient and removal of waste products occurs [53]. Moreover, syncytiotrophoblast have an endocrine function characterized by production of human chorionic gonadotrophin (hCG) regulated by progesterone [50]. Besides, those cells also secrete a variant of growth hormone (GH), human placental lactogen (hPL), insulin-like growth factor I (IGF-I) and endothelial growth factor [50,53]. On the other hand, cytotrophoblasts (or Langhans´cells) are continually differentiating into syncytiotrophoblast. In addition, this layer also may synthesize hCG [54]. There is a trophoblastic basement membrane supporting these two layers, cytotrophoblast and syncythiotrophoblast. This membrane forms the physical separation of those layers with the stromal core villi, a structure formed by connective tissue where the fetal vessels are immersed.

In the placenta, the blood vessels constitute the largest component among the structures creating the cotyledons. These vessels are an intricate network coming from and going to the fetus. In fact, placental vessels constitute a continuous circulatory system with the fetal cardiovascular system. In the placenta, the veins are conducting oxygenated blood toward the fetus, whereas the arteries contain deoxygenated blood toward the placenta. Anatomically, from the umbilical cord to the deep in the placental cotyledons, the umbilical arteries and veins branch themselves to form chorionic arteries and vein, respectively, over fetal surface of the term placenta, and those branches subdivide themselves before entering into the villi. The chorionic arteries generally cross over the chorionic veins [53]. Likewise other vascular beds, in the placenta the veins are more elastic, exhibit high capacity and a miniscule layer of both smooth muscle cells and adventitia compared to arteries; which in turn are vessels that offer a high resistance. These characteristics, especially those observed in the umbilical cord, have been used for functional non invasive studies, like Doppler, in order to analyze the status of the feto-placental circulation. Finally, and similar to any other tissue, the placenta blood vessels are lined by the endothelium. In fact, these cells are obligatory constituent of blood microvessels [55]. The endothelial cells are supported by a basal membrane and pericytes, both of them involved in vessel permeability and integrity, and importantly in the endothelium differentiation [56].

In GDM, it has been reported macroscopical and histological alterations in the term placenta. For instance, placental size and placental weight [57] are elevated in GDM, which produce a reduced fetal/placental weight ratio compared to normal pregnancy [58,59], that means, the placenta growth is even higher than fetal growth. On the other hand, regarding studies, in syncytiotrophoblast from diabetes during pregnancy, have shown functional alteration in this cell type. Thus, it has been described an increase in the number of cytotrophoblast identified by number of nuclei [60], high fibrin deposit over syncytiotrophoblast and hyperplasia of cytotrophoblast [59,61,62], whose in turn may be related with the enhancement of the thickness of syncytial basement membranes in GDM compared to normal pregnancy [63]. Moreover, using functional studies of syncytiotrophoblast microvillous membrane vesicles, Jansson and collages [64] showed non-changes in the glucose transport in samples from GDM. Contrarily, other reports showed reduced glucose uptake and glucose utilization [65], as well as low expression of glucose transporter type 1 (GLUT1) and 3 (GLUT 3) in placentas from GDM compared with non-diabetic controls [66]. Other alterations in the throphoblastic cells from GDM were low expression of serotonin transporter (SERT) and receptors (5-HT2A) [67], as well as high activity of amino acid transporter system A [68]. Nevertheless, it has been reported a high expression of inducible nitric oxide synthase (iNOS) in the whole placenta but mainly in the trophoblastic cells using immunohistochemistry in GDM [69], a phenomena that may be correlated with high nitric oxide synthesis [24] and nitrative stress [70] observed in placentas from GDM.

In addition, it has been reported high level of degenerative lesions such as fibrinoid necrosis and vascular lesions like chorangiosis, as well as elevated signs of villous immaturity and presence of nucleated fetal erithrocytes in placentas from GDM compared to normal pregnancy [58]. In particular, the presence of microscopic signs of villous immaturity (i.e., hypervascularization), as well as the presence of fetal erithrocytes and microscopic signs of ischemia [71] may suggest that placenta in GDM exhibits a high metabolic demand and oxygen consumption, which in turn, it is generating a "relative hypoxic" status in the fetus. Thus, it has been reported in GDM that the elevation of plasma glucose in the umbilical vein is associated with reduced oxygen saturation and oxygen content, as well as a significant increase of lactate concentration compared with normal pregnancy [59]. Interestingly, these changes were not observed in the umbilical artery, suggesting high placental oxygen consumption in GDM, which may generate a compensatory response in the placenta itself. In fact, as it will be described later in this chapter (see below), elevated vessel formation (i.e., angiogenesis) has been described in the placenta from GDM [18,72,73,74,75], which may explain the high placental "mass" observed in this disease. Therefore, placental alteration in GDM includes changes in the transport of nutrients (such as amino acid), enhanced blood formation and glucose consumption that may generate a "relative hypoxic" status. Unfortunately, all this findings are described in term placenta; therefore, non-invasive test such as Doppler will offer more clinically relevant information regarding fetal status and feto-placental circulation before delivery.

6. Placental blood flow and GDM

One of the non-invasive techniques used widely to estimate the blood flow in the feto-placental circulation is Ultrasound and Doppler. In this regard, the normal flow between 24 and 29 weeks of gestation in the umbilical vein is 443 ± 91.6 ml/min and normalized to fetal weight is 131.0 ± 19.8 (mL/kg/min) [76]. Moreover, the absence of end-diastolic blood flow before 36 weeks gestation is utilized clinically as indicator of fetal distress such hypoxia and acidosis [77] and this indicator is also associated to growth restriction [78].

Wharton's jelly area is surrounding the two arteries and the vein in the umbilical cord, and this jelly has a protective role for preventing interruption of flow by compression or twisting caused by fetal movement [79]. Wharton's jelly area can be determined by subtraction of umbilical cord area and total vessels area (arteries and vein), and interestingly it is significant correlated with gestational age and fetal anthropometric parameters [79,80], and also it has been described that alterations in this parameter are associated to hypertensive disorders, fetal distress, gestational diabetes and fetal growth restriction [80].

Doppler studies in umbilical vein from GDM have shown no changes neither in the pulsatile index value in the umbilical artery nor in the mean total umbilical venous flow in fetus exposed to GDM compared to normal pregnancy [81]. Interestingly, large for gestational-age fetus showed an increase in the total umbilical venous flow, suggesting that high placental flow toward the fetus may be associated with macrosomia. Moreover in macrosomic fetus without diabetes, it has shown an increase in the umbilical vein blood flow associated with high systolic velocity in the splenic, superior mesenteric, cerebral and umbilical arteries [82], suggesting an increased fetal perfusion especially in the liver. The underling mechanisms for this redistribution in the blood flow are unclear, but considering that GDM increases the synthesis of nitric oxide in human umbilical vein endothelial cells [83], it is feasible to speculate that a overall vasodilatation in the pre-hepatic and hepatic circulation would be taken part in this process. Taken these evidences into account, it is feasible that elevated feto-placental blood flow and hyperglycemia would be responsible for macrosomia in GDM. However, the underling mechanisms of this relationship are part of ongoing investigations, and may include the synthesis and secretion of vasoactive substances from the fetal-placental endothelium, as it will be discussed in the next section.

a. Mechanism of vascular tone regulation in the placenta during GD: Role of endothelial cells

Endothelium in the feto-placental circulation is involved in a series of specific mechanism aimed to ensure the input of nutrients and oxygen to the fetus. These mechanisms include; maintenance of physiological barrier, regulation of vascular tone and angiogenesis. Importantly, feto-placental endothelium forms an uninterrupted tissue that will be extended until fetal circulation, where it is exposed to the same metabolic and hormonal medium than endothelium of the fetus itself [84]. Moreover, since the lack of innervation of the placenta, the regulation of vascular tone is mainly dependent on endothelial cells-mediated synthesis and release of several vasoactive substances including, nitric oxide (NO), prostacyclin, thromboxane, endothelial derived hyperpolarizing factor (EDHF), adenosine, mono or di or tri monophosphate of adenosine (AMP, ADP, ATP), among others [85,86,87]. These characteristics are summarized in the Figure 1, where it also described some functional alterations observed in GDM. On the other hand, there are emerging evidences showing that endothelial cells are able to dedifferentiate into mesenchymal cells, via a process called endothelial-to-mesenchymal transition (EndMT) [88,89], which in fact is related with the capacity of the endothelium to migrate away from the vessel-lining and colonize other tissues where dedifferentiation may occur in order to recover the particular capacity required by the invaded tissue. Additionally, endothelial cells exhibit a capacity to form new vessels (i.e., angiogenesis) via enhancement of its proliferation and migration toward the tissue where it would be required [90]. Both, dedifferentiation and vessel formation are mechanisms controlled by extracellular signals that are sensed by membrane receptors in the endothelium. Among others, transforming growth factor-β (TGF- β), VEGF, extracellular nucleosides (i.e., adenosine, ATP) have been related with endothelial function. Therefore, it is not surprising that endothelium exhibits a specialized function according with its cell localization and mainly according with the extracellular medium where they are seeded [91,92,93]. Taken these evidences into account, endothelium has been considered as a specialized endocrine organ which is able to control the vascular homeostasis in normal conditions; and its malfunctioning (i.e., endothelial dysfunction) has been related with several cardiovascular diseases, including hypertension and diabetes [86,87,94].

Human placenta is an unique source of endothelial cells for studying functional differences considering vessel distribution. Thus, it has been estimated that >70% of the placental tissue is constituted by blood vessels and length of fetal capillaries would be covering an area of 223 miles [91]. In addition, since autonomic control of the vascular resistance will not be part of the mechanisms for controlling blood distribution, endothelial cells are responsible for

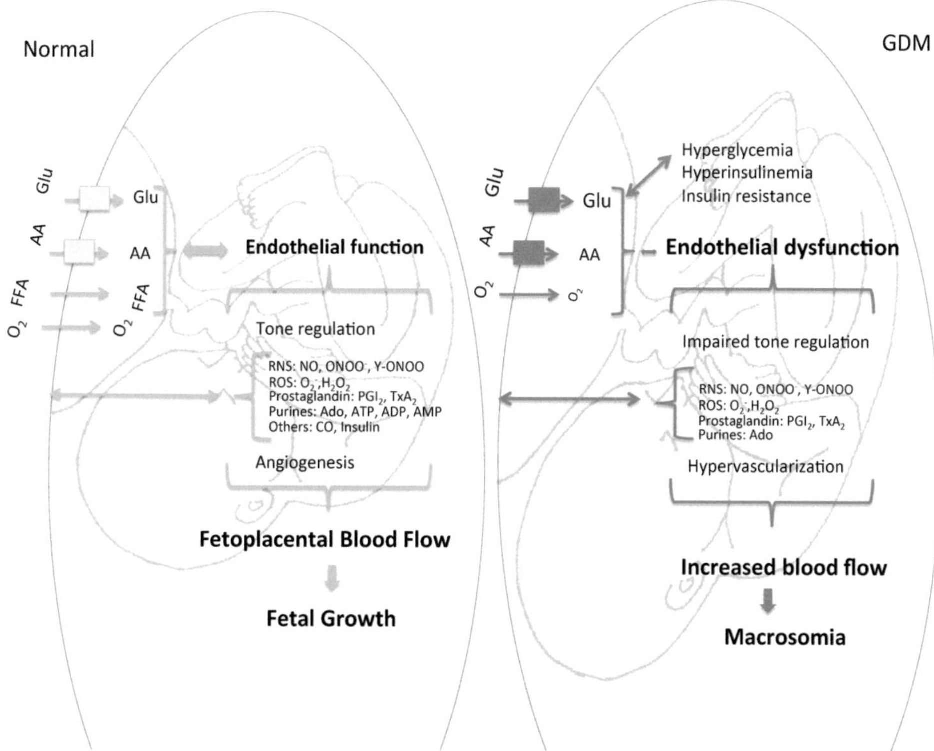

Figure 1. Role of feto-placental endothelial function in fetal growth during normal pregnancy and gestational diabetes. In normal pregnancy (Normal), the nutrients that includes glucose (Glu), amino acids (AA) are incorporated to the feto-placental circulation via specific transporters (boxes) whereas liposoluble molecules such as free fatty acids (FFA) and oxygen (O_2) pass through by simple diffusion (i.e., without transporters). These transport mechanisms are in a perfect equilibrium between demand and consumption, and they are highly dependent on the appropriated endothelial function in the placental vascular bed. In turn, endothelial function include: 1) the synthesis and release of vasoactive molecules including reactive nitrogen species (RNS) such as nitric oxide (NO), peroxinitrite (ONOO) and nitrotyrosine (Y-ONOO); reactive oxygen species (ROS), such as superoxide (O_2^-) and hydrogen peroxide (H_2O_2); prostaglandin such as prostacyclin (PGI_2) and thromboxane A_2; purines including adenosine (Ado), adenosine tri-di-or mono phosphate (ATP, ADP, AMP, respectively); and others factors such as carbon monoxide (CO), or insulin. 2) Capacity for vessel formation form pre-existing vessels (i.e., angiogenesis). Both, vasomotor and angiogenic properties are modulating the fetoplacental blood flow continually by a cross talking between placenta and fetus. On the other hand, there is an increase in the glucose level in the maternal circulation in gestational diabetes mellitus (GDM), which is transported to the feto-placental circulation generating and stated of hyperglycemia, hyperinsulinemia and insulin resistance. In turn this high glucose uptake may generate elevated oxygen consumption due to high metabolism. This elevation in the glucose metabolism in the placenta would generate an endothelial dysfunction characterized by elevation in RNS, ROS, prostaglandin and purine concentration in the feto-placental circulation, which consequently affects the tone regulation in the placenta. Moreover, relative hypoxic condition in GDM, may trigger an pro-angiogenic response generating a condition of hypervascularization in the placenta and therefore creating a vicious circle. Those alterations would be related with increased blood flow observed in Doppler studies. Finally, this high input of nutrients and elevated circulation will be responsible for macrosomia in GDM.

supplying this lack. Moreover, in human placenta, several studies have been shown that endothelium exhibits morphological and functional differences according to the vascular bed where they are coming from [84,87,91,92]. Some of these differences have been described in recently published reviewers [84,87]. For instance and similarly to the pulmonary circulation in the adult, the feto-placental endothelium has a particular distribution. The veins transport oxygen and nutrients whereas the arteries contain de-oxygenated blood coming from the fetus. In terms of endothelial-derived vasomotor response, it has been described that acute hypoxia in the placental microvessels generates constriction [95], whereas this challenge generates augmentation of the umbilical blood flow [96]; this phenomenon is attributed to blood redistribution such occurs in the pulmonary circulation. Additionally, it has been also described in samples from umbilical endothelial cells exposed to hypoxia, that the one from the artery has a different response (i.e., high activation of endothelial nitric oxide synthase, without changes in arginase-2) than endothelium vein (i.e, low activation of eNOS, associated to high levels of arginase-2) [97]. In addition, HUVEC (i.e, macrovascular endothelium) showed a reduced synthesis of angiotensin II, thromboxane B_2, 6-keto-prostaglandin, and endothelin 1,2 compared to placental microvascular endothelial cells (hPMEC) [91]. Other functional differences occurred in the capacity for generating new vessels (i.e., angiogenesis). Thus, placental microvascular placental cells exposed to VEGF or placental growth factor (PlGF) showed a high mitogen response compared to HUVEC [91], a phenomena associated with high expression of VEGF receptor 1 (VEGFR-1) and 2 (VEGFR-2) [98] in this cell type. In addition, using feto-placental tissue it has been described that several genes related with angiogenic response are preferentially expressed in microvascular than macrovascular endothelium [86,87,91,92]. In this regards, studying functional differences between HUVEC and hPMEC, preliminary results (see Figure 2) showed that the tube formation in matrigel is faster in hPMEC than HUVEC, corroborating differences in the VEGF expression.

Several studies have reported dysfunction of feto-placental endothelium during GDM [18,74, 75,84,86,91,93,99]. In this regard, one of the most studied pathway in our group is the L-adenosine/L-arginine/NO (i.e., ALANO pathway) [100]. For instances, it has been described that L-arginine transport- mainly via the cationic aminoacid transport type 1 (CAT-1) - is increased in HUVEC from GDM [87,100,101,102]. Besides this alteration, it has been described high expression and activity of endothelial nitric oxide synthase (eNOS) [24,103] as well as iNOS [69] in both umbilical and placental endothelium from GDM. This enhancement would produce a high synthesis and release of NO [20,24], which in turn has been related with a nitrative status in the placenta and umbilical cord from this disease [104,105]. In addition, NO reduces the expression of adenosine transport via hENT-1 [83] and may generate augmentation in the extracellular level of adenosine in umbilical blood [106]. In turn, adenosine activates adenosine receptors (AR) spreading the vascular effects of NO in the feto-placental circulation in both vascular tone regulation [87,100,102] and promoting angiogenesis (see below). Therefore, it is feasible to speculate that the elevation in NO synthesis during GDM may explain the augmented umbilical flow observed in macrosomic fetuses [82].

b. GD and oxidative stress in the placenta

As detailed above, GDM has been associated with impaired placental development characterized by high placental weights and low ratios between fetal and placental weights [107]. Remarkably, one of the cellular mechanisms associated with the etiology of these

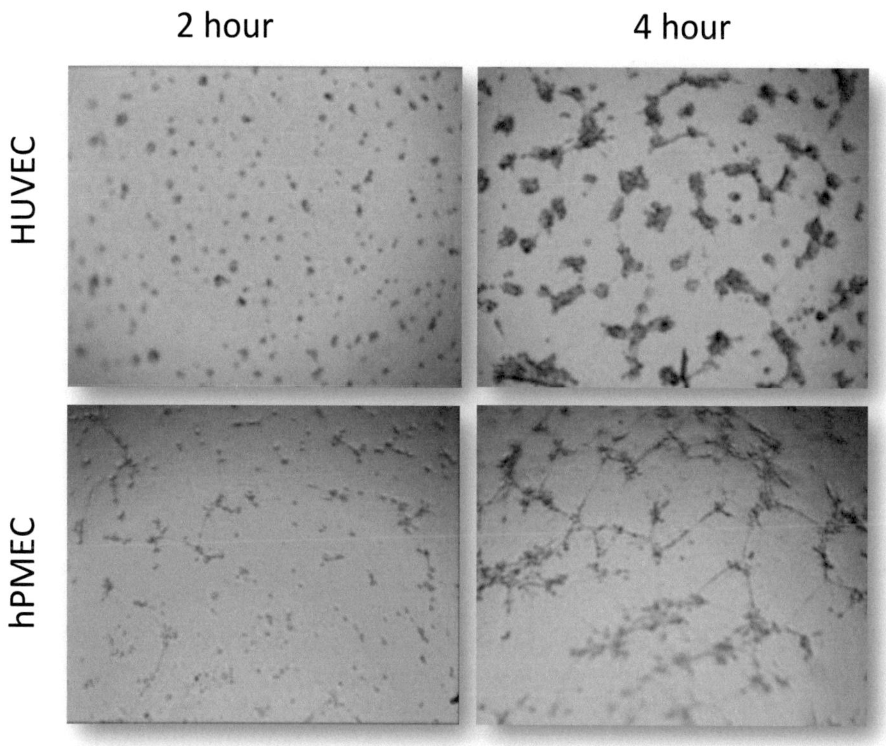

Figure 2. Differential capacity in the angiogenic ability of the fetal endothelium. Representative images of tube formation assay in matrigel using primary cultured human umbilical vein endothelial cells (HUVEC; i.e., macrovascular) and human placental microvascular endothelial cells (hPMEC; i.e., microvascular) isolated from normal pregnancy. After overnight serum deprivation, cells were seeded on the matrigel in a different number since 10 x 10^3 to 30 x 10^3 cells/ml prepared in culture medium (M199) without serum. In the images is presented only HUVEC that were seeded at 30 x 10^3 and hPMEC that were seeded at 10 x 10^3. Those cells were maintained in culture under standard conditions (5% CO_2, 37°C) during 0, 1, 2, 3 and 4 hours and cells were photographed. As indicated in the pictures, hPMEC exhibit a more rapid response for tube formation under our culture condition and require lesser quantity of cells than HUVEC, suggesting a differential physiological role of these cells in the fetal circulation.

changes is the oxidative stress, which is related with an imbalance between the synthesis of reactive oxygen and nitrogen species (ROS and RNS, respectively) and the activity of antioxidant enzymes. The most relevant free radicals are superoxide ($O_2^{\bullet-}$) in the ROS group; and nitric oxide (NO) and peroxinitrite ($ONOO^-$) in the RNS group. In addition, considering the diffusion distance, NO can diffuse from endothelial cells to smooth muscle cells, whereas $O_2^{\bullet-}$ and $ONOO^-$ would have actions within the cells where they were synthesized [70]. The main sources of $O_2^{\bullet-}$ in the placenta include the mitochondrial electron transport chain, xanthine oxidase, NADPH oxidase and uncoupled endothelial NO synthase (eNOS) [21,108], whereas the main source of NO are the endothelial and inducible NO synthases (eNOS and iNOS, respectively)[70,85].

The oxidative stress is an inherent condition of pregnancy related with the increasing metabolism of fetal and utero-placental tissues, which results in a continue delivery of oxygen –and nutrients- toward the developing fetus. In fact, it has been described that the elevation in the normal metabolic rate of feto-placental tissues increases the oxidative stress in the placental [109]. Moreover, in placental tissue from early pregnancy has been determined a higher activity of NADPH oxidase; therefore, the synthesis of $O_2^{\bullet -}$ is more marked at the end of the first trimester than the activity in term placental tissue [110]. On the other hand, studies using samples obtained from patients with GDM showed that there is an increased activity of xanthine oxidase (XO) and a decreased activity of catalase in maternal plasma, umbilical cord plasma and placental tissue [111]. These findings showed that there is an impairment of antioxidant defenses in the placenta and blood from mother and newborn, which might be related with the high mortality and morbidity in both mother and newborn observed during GDM pregnancies. In addition, placental tissues from GDM exhibited a decreased response to oxidative stress induced by hypoxanthine plus XO, as was reflected by a reduced levels of catalase and glutathione peroxidase (GPx) after exposition to the pro-oxidative challenge, suggesting that placental tissues from GDM would be exposed to damage in an oxidative environment [112].

The hallmark of diabetes is hyperglycemia whose condition has been associated with increases of synthesis of ROS and RNS in tissues and cell cultures from umbilical cord and placenta. There is an increase of ROS levels in HUVEC exposed to high extracellular concentration of D-glucose mediated by activity of NADPH oxidase in a mechanism that involved a decrease of NO bioavailability and increases of vascular reactivity in umbilical veins [21,113]. In HUVEC, it has been described that the higher increase in the NADPH oxidase-mediated ROS induced by high concentration of D-glucose, the higher NO synthesis mediated by eNOS [21,113]. Considering the reaction rate between $O_2^{\bullet -}$ and NO, it is highly probable that the hyperglycemic condition induces the synthesis of $ONOO^-$; therefore, it contributes to the development of endothelial dysfunction in umbilical cord and placenta. Long-term incubation (7-14 days) of HUVEC with high concentration of high D-glucose increases the expression of regulatory subunits of NADPH oxidase $p67^{phox}$ and $p47^{phox}$ [114], whereas 24 hours incubation of the same cell type with high D-glucose increases the expression of the catalytic subunits NOX2 and NOX4 [113]. Thus, an increased expression and activity of NADPH oxidase would be a hallmark of HUVEC exposed to hyperglycemic, suggesting that the same phenomenon would be present in GDM.

On the other hand, recently data has been shown that in trophoblastic cells ACH-3P, incubated at 21 % oxygen and under normoglycemic condition, increases ROS levels after 3 days. Interestingly, ACH-3P cells treated (3 days) with high extracellular concentration of D-glucose increases the ROS levels only in cells exposed to lower percentage of oxygen (2.5 %). In fact, in ACH-3P cells, hyperglycemic conditions increase the mitochondrial $O_2^{\bullet -}$ levels. Therefore, this study is showing that ROS production in normoglycemia is oxygen-dependent but oxygen-independent in hyperglycemia. The mechanism involved in this phenomenon could involve the increase of expression and/or activity of oxidant enzymes present in placental tissue [115].

In summary, there is an imbalance in the control of redox cellular status in pathological conditions related with increases blood concentrations of molecules that induce oxidative stress, like GDM and hyperglycemia, probably due to a higher expression of oxidant enzymes like NADPH oxidase, XO and deregulation of metabolic pathways of NO.

c. Placental angiogenesis and GDM

Angiogenesis is a general term that involves the physiological process leading to growth of new blood vessels from a pre-formed one. This is a vital process involved in embryological growth, tissue development, would healing of damaged tissues and in the context of this chapter is a crucial process for placental development and fetal growth during normal and GDM. In this regard, as it has been remarked before, macrosomia, present in GDM, has been associated to increased nutrient delivery toward the fetus, a phenomenon that may be related with increased blood flow due to vasodilatation of placental vessels [100]. Moreover, angiogenesis in the placenta is also controlling blood flow toward the fetus, and in fact, the vessel formation proceed to any vascular function, this process (i.e., angiogenesis) has been studied as one of the underling mechanism for explaining macrosomia in GDM [116,117,118,119]. Thus, placentas from GDM exhibits elevated number of redundant capillary connections per villi, compared to normal pregnancy, suggesting a more intense capillary branching [120]. Moreover, there are increased placental capillary length, branching and surface area that have been reported in women with type 1 [121], pre-gestational and gestational diabetes [18,74], as well as elevated number of terminal villi and capillaries in women with hyperglycemia [73]. In addition, it has been reported that glycemic control was significant correlated with capillary surface area and capillary volume in women with pre-gestational diabetes [117]. Moreover, it is well known that diabetes is associated with increased angiogenic response in some specific tissues such as eye, where hyperglycemia can lead to retinopathy [122]. Nevertheless, it has been shown that GDM is associated to reduction in the circulating endothelial progenitor cells (EPC), in mother and fetus [123,124] a phenomenon that was linking with reduced capacity for recovering endothelial dysfunction in GDM.

Associated mechanism behind increased placental angiogenesis in GDM may be related to the pro-angiogenic effect of hyperglycemia [125], which in turn triggers an enhancement in the placental synthesis and release of VEGF, as well as the expression of VEGF receptors (VEGFR) and nitric oxide production [18]. Thus, it has been shown that the placentas from women with hyperglycemia exhibited high levels of VEGF and VEGF receptor 2 (VEGFR-2) but reduced expression of VEGF receptor 1 (VEGFR-1) [73]. Furthermore, it has been reported elevated placental levels of VEGFR-1 mainly in vascular and throphoblastic cells in women with GDM [73,126]. Also, alteration in VEGF-VEGFRs expression has been described in women with type 1 diabetes [18,61,75,127]. Thus, the increased secretion and activity of VEGF may explain hypervascularization observed in placentas from DGM [58,71]

On the other hand, increased placental angiogenic response may also be related with hyperinsulinemia present in GDM. In this regard, it has been described that insulin activates at least two types of insulin receptors (IR), type A (IR-A, associated with a mitogenic phenotype) and type B (IR-B, associated with a metabolic phenotype), which are elevated in both HUVEC [24] and hPMEC [106], respectively. This particular localization of insulin receptors in feto-placental endothelium, may be linked with the differential proliferative capacity of endothelial cells, since insulin increases the expression of several genes related with angiogenesis (i.e., EFNB2) and vascularization (i.e., EPAS1) mainly in placental derived endothelium [128], therefore is feasible that functional clustering of insulin-regulated genes in this cell type may promote their mitotic potential.

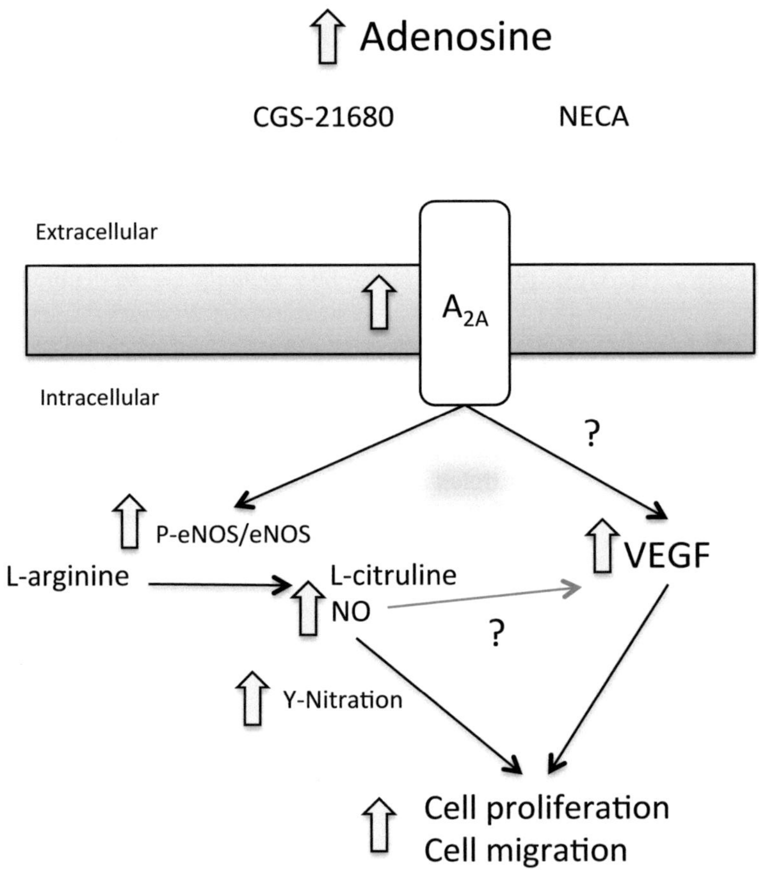

Figure 3. Potential role of A_{2A}AR/NO/VEGF signaling pathway in the cell migration and proliferation during gestational diabetes mellitus. In human umbilical vein endothelial cells (HUVEC), adenosine or adenosine receptor agonists (CGS-21680 or NECA) activate A_{2A} adenosine receptor (A_{2A}) and trigger the activation (i.e., phosphorylation in serine 1177, p-eNOS) of endothelial nitric oxide synthase (eNOS), without changes in total eNOS, which in turn is associated with elevation of nitric oxide synthesis (NO) and nitration of tyrosine residues (Y-nitration), enhancing the synthesis of vascular endothelial growth factor (VEGF) and then this activation generates cell migration and proliferation. It is unknown (?) the mechanism(s) associated with the regulation of expression of VEGF mediated by A_{2A}/NO signaling pathway. Preliminary results in our laboratory suggest that gestational diabetes mellitus (GDM) is associated with elevation of adenosine extracellular levels and high activation and expression of A_{2A} adenosine receptor characterized by high (⇧) eNOS activation, NO formation and Y-nitration whose are associated to enhancement of cell proliferation and migration and finally it would be occasioned elevated placental angiogenesis characteristic of this disease.

Another potential pathway, involved in the increase of placental angiogenesis during GDM, may be the ALANO pathway described before [100]. In this regard, we have previously proposed that a dysfunction in this pathway is taken part in the physiopathology of reduced placental angiogenesis in pre-eclampsia [129]. Therefore, it is feasible that the converse may be occurring in GDM. Considering this idea, preliminary results have shown that HUVEC from gestational diabetes was associated with high expression of A_{2A} and A_{2B} adenosine receptors (AR) (~6 and ~2-fold, respectively). Moreover, CGS-21680 (A_{2A}AR selective agonist) and NECA (AR non selective agonist) increase (~2 and 2.5-fold) cell proliferation in both gestational diabetes and normal pregnancies; an effect that was blocked by ZM-241385 (A_{2A}AR selective antagonist) only in normal pregnancies. Interestingly, a shift in the curve of ZM-241385 by inhibiting the stimulatory effect of CGS-21680 was observed in diabetic pregnancies compared with normal pregnancies (calculated *Ki* 1.3 ± 0.2 and 12.8 ± 3.4 nM, respectively). Interestingly, co-incubation with L-NAME (NOS non-selective antagonist) blocked the CGS-21680-mediated proliferation in both normal and pathological pregnancies. Therefore, this results suggest that A_{2A}AR stimulation increases cell proliferation in gestational diabetes through an intracellular pathway dependent of NO synthesis. Remarkable, these results also suggested that a posttranslational modification in A_{2A}AR could be involved in the reduced affinity to ZM-241385 in GDM (Escudero A and Escudero C, unpublished results) (see Figure 3).

7. Concluding remarks

As detailed above, intrauterine exposure to diabetes has been associated with high risk of diabetes, obesity, as well as cardiovascular disease in the offspring. Although the genetic component is hard to discard, the general agreement is that intrauterine exposition allows the "transmission" of diabetes to the offspring. Several mechanisms have been proposed in order to understand the relationship between maternal GDM and the risk of metabolic and cardiovascular disease in the offspring. In this review, we have highlighted some information regarding the potential role of placental dysfunction and particularly placental endothelial dysfunction as one of the mechanisms linking with fetal programming in GDM. This relationship is not arbitrary because it may constitute the basis for explaining other pregnancy diseases such as growth restriction or pre-eclampsia, where the same alteration, might explain the predisposition that the children "exposed" to those diseases could develop metabolic or cardiovascular disease later in life. Therefore, if we consider this phenomenon (i.e., endothelial dysfunction) is a "normal" response in front of intrauterine stressful conditions, such as GDM or intrauterine growth restriction or pre-eclampsia; it would offer an opportunity to plan clinical strategies addressing to evaluate and control endothelial function as soon as the babies, exposed to those diseases, have been born. Finally, a general recommendation would be that it is necessary to establish a consensus for diagnosis of GDM. This is particularly important because hyperglycemia would be one of the most affecting factors involved in the endothelial dysfunction and fetal programming.

Abbreviations

Adenosine receptor (AR), Cationic aminoacid transport type 1 (CAT-1), Diabetes in Pregnancy Study Group (IADPSG), Diabetes mellitus type 2 (DMT2), Endothelial derived hyperpolarizing factor (EDHF), Endothelial nitric oxide synthase (eNOS), Endothelial-to-mesenchymal transition (EndMT), Equilibrative Nucleside Transport type 1 (ENT-1), Gestational diabetes mellitus (GDM), Glucose transporter (GLUT), Glutathione peroxidase (GPX), Growth hormone (GH), Human chorionic gonadotrophin (hCG), Human placental lactogen (hPl), Human placental microvascular endothelial cells (hPMEC), Human umbilical vein endothelial cells (HUVEC), Hyperglycemia and Adverse Pregnancy Outcomes (HAPO), Inducible NOS (iNOS), nitric oxide (NO), Insulin-dependent diabetes (IDDM), Insulin-like growth factor I (IGF-I), Large for gestational age (LGA), Oral glucose tolerance test (OGTT), Reactive nitrogen species (RNS), Reactive oxygen species (ROS), Serotonin transporter (SERT), Transforming growth factor-β (TGF- β), Vascular endothelial growth factor (VEGF), Vascular endothelial growth factor (VEGF), VEGF receptor (VEGFR), Xanthine oxidase (XO).

Acknowledgements

Supported by Fondo Nacional de Desarrollo Científico y Tecnológico (FONDECYT 1110977, 1120928, 11110059, 1100684), Comisión Nacional de Investigación en Ciencia y Tecnología (CONICYT PIA Anillos ACT-73, AT-24100210), Chile. Conicyt 79112027. Direccion de Investigacion, DIUBB 122109 GI/EF. The authors thank the research staff belongs to the Group of Investigation in Tumoral Angiogenesis (GIANT) and the Vascular Physiology Laboratory, Universidad del Bio Bio, Chile. Authors also thank to the Hospital Clinico Universidad Católica de Chile and Hospital Clinico Herminda Martin from Chillan labour ward staff for the supply of placenta, and the staff at the Cellular and Molecular Physiology Laboratory (CMPL) at PUC, Chile. We would like to thanks to Mr. Cristian Celis for editing this manuscript.

Author details

Carlos Escudero[1*], Marcelo González[2], Jesenia Acurio[1], Francisco Valenzuela[1] and Luis Sobrevia[3]

*Address all correspondence to: cescudero@ubiobio.cl, sobrevia@med.puc.cl

1 Vascular Physiology Laboratory, Group of Investigation in Tumor Angiogenesis (GIANT), Department of Basic Sciences, University of Bío-Bío, Chillán, Chile

2 Vascular Physiology Laboratory, Department of Physiology, University of Concepcion, Concepcion, Chile

3 Cellular and Molecular Physiology Laboratory (CMPL), Division of Obstetrics and Gynecology, Faculty of Medicine, School of Medicine, Pontificia Universidad Católica de Chile, Santiago, Chile

References

[1] Stanley, K, Fraser, R, & Bruce, C. (1998). Physiological changes in insulin resistance in human pregnancy: longitudinal study with the hyperinsulinaemic euglycaemic clamp technique. Br J Obstet Gynaecol , 105, 756-759.

[2] Wendland, E. M, Torloni, M. R, Falavigna, M, Trujillo, J, Dode, M. A, et al. (2012). Gestational diabetes and pregnancy outcomes--a systematic review of the World Health Organization (WHO) and the International Association of Diabetes in Pregnancy Study Groups (IADPSG) diagnostic criteria. BMC Pregnancy Childbirth 12: 23.

[3] Alberti, K. G, & Zimmet, P. Z. (1998). Definition, diagnosis and classification of diabetes mellitus and its complications. Part 1: diagnosis and classification of diabetes mellitus provisional report of a WHO consultation. Diabet Med , 15, 539-553.

[4] Metzger, B. E, Lowe, L. P, Dyer, A. R, Trimble, E. R, Chaovarindr, U, et al. (2008). Hyperglycemia and adverse pregnancy outcomes. The N Engl J Med , 358, 1991-2002.

[5] Veeraswamy, S, Vijayam, B, Gupta, V. K, & Kapur, A. (2012). Gestational diabetes: The public health relevance and approach. Diabetes Res Clin Pract. , 97, 350-358.

[6] Girgis, C. M, Gunton, J. E, & Cheung, N. W. (2012). The influence of ethnicity on the development of type 2 diabetes mellitus in women with gestational diabetes: a prospective study and review of the literature. ISRN Endocrinol 2012: 341638.

[7] Sacks, D. A, Hadden, D. R, Maresh, M, Deerochanawong, C, Dyer, A. R, et al. (2012). Frequency of gestational diabetes mellitus at collaborating centers based on IADPSG consensus panel-recommended criteria: the Hyperglycemia and Adverse Pregnancy Outcome (HAPO) Study. Diabetes Care , 35, 526-528.

[8] Dabelea, D, Snell-bergeon, J. K, Hartsfield, C. L, Bischoff, K. J, Hamman, R. F, et al. (2005). Increasing prevalence of gestational diabetes mellitus (GDM) over time and by birth cohort: Kaiser Permanente of Colorado GDM Screening Program. Diabetes Care , 28, 579-584.

[9] Anna, V, Van Der Ploeg, H. P, Cheung, N. W, Huxley, R. R, & Bauman, A. E. (2008). Sociodemographic correlates of the increasing trend in prevalence of gestational diabetes mellitus in a large population of women between 1995 and 2005. Diabetes Care , 31, 2288-2293.

[10] Buchanan, T. A, Xiang, A. H, & Page, K. A. (2012). Gestational diabetes mellitus: risks and management during and after pregnancy. Nat Rev Endocrinol , 8, 639-649.

[11] Homko, C, Sivan, E, Chen, X, Reece, E. A, & Boden, G. (2001). Insulin secretion during and after pregnancy in patients with gestational diabetes mellitus. J Clin Endocrinol Metab , 86, 568-573.

[12] Lenzen, S. (2008). The mechanisms of alloxan- and streptozotocin-induced diabetes. Diabetologia , 51, 216-226.

[13] Prior, R. L, & Smith, S. B. (1983). Role of insulin in regulating amino acid metabolism in normal and alloxan-diabetic cattle. J Nutr , 113, 1016-1031.

[14] Khan, K. S, Wojdyla, D, Say, L, Gulmezoglu, A. M, & Van Look, P. F. (2006). WHO analysis of causes of maternal death: a systematic review. Lancet , 367, 1066-1074.

[15] Gluckman, P. D, & Hanson, M. A. (2004). Living with the past: evolution, development, and patterns of disease. Science , 305, 1733-1736.

[16] Hanson, M. A, & Gluckman, P. D. (2008). Developmental origins of health and disease: new insights. Basic Clin Pharmacol Toxicol , 102, 90-93.

[17] Ericsson, A, Saljo, K, Sjostrand, E, Jansson, N, Prasad, P. D, et al. (2007). Brief hyperglycaemia in the early pregnant rat increases fetal weight at term by stimulating placental growth and affecting placental nutrient transport. J Physiol , 581, 1323-1332.

[18] Leach, L, Taylor, A, & Sciota, F. (2009). Vascular dysfunction in the diabetic placenta: causes and consequences. J Anat , 215, 69-76.

[19] Guzman-gutierrez, E, Abarzua, F, Belmar, C, Nien, J. K, Ramirez, M. A, et al. (2011). Functional link between adenosine and insulin: a hypothesis for fetoplacental vascular endothelial dysfunction in gestational diabetes. Curr Vasc Pharmacol , 9, 750-762.

[20] Westermeier, F, Puebla, C, Vega, J. L, Farias, M, Escudero, C, et al. (2009). Equilibrative nucleoside transporters in fetal endothelial dysfunction in diabetes mellitus and hyperglycaemia. Curr Vasc Pharmacol , 7, 435-449.

[21] Sobrevia, L, & Gonzalez, M. (2009). A role for insulin on L-arginine transport in fetal endothelial dysfunction in hyperglycaemia. Curr Vasc Pharmacol , 7, 467-474.

[22] Gonzalez, M, Gallardo, V, Rodriguez, N, Salomon, C, Westermeier, F, et al. (2011). Insulin-stimulated L-arginine transport requires SLC7A1 gene expression and is associated with human umbilical vein relaxation. J Cell Physiol , 226, 2916-2924.

[23] Jones, H. N, Jansson, T, & Powell, T. L. (2010). Full-length adiponectin attenuates insulin signaling and inhibits insulin-stimulated amino Acid transport in human primary trophoblast cells. Diabetes , 59, 1161-1170.

[24] Westermeier, F, Salomon, C, Gonzalez, M, Puebla, C, Guzman-gutierrez, E, et al. (2011). Insulin restores gestational diabetes mellitus-reduced adenosine transport involving differential expression of insulin receptor isoforms in human umbilical vein endothelium. Diabetes , 60, 1677-1687.

[25] Simeoni, U, & Barker, D. J. (2009). Offspring of diabetic pregnancy: long-term outcomes. Semin Fetal Neonatal Med , 14, 119-124.

[26] Barker, D. J, Winter, P. D, Osmond, C, Margetts, B, & Simmonds, S. J. (1989). Weight in infancy and death from ischaemic heart disease. Lancet , 2, 577-580.

[27] Rees, S, & Inder, T. (2005). Fetal and neonatal origins of altered brain development. Early Hum Dev , 81, 753-761.

[28] Glover, V. (2011). Annual Research Review: Prenatal stress and the origins of psychopathology: an evolutionary perspective. J Child Psychol Psychiatry , 52, 356-367.

[29] Hanley, B, Dijane, J, Fewtrell, M, Grynberg, A, Hummel, S, et al. (2010). Metabolic imprinting, programming and epigenetics- a review of present priorities and future opportunities. Br J Nutr 104 Suppl 1: S, 1-25.

[30] Nuyt, A. M. (2008). Mechanisms underlying developmental programming of elevated blood pressure and vascular dysfunction: evidence from human studies and experimental animal models. Clin Sci (Lond) , 114, 1-17.

[31] Davis, E. F, Newton, L, Lewandowski, A. J, Lazdam, M, Kelly, B. A, et al. (2012). Preeclampsia and offspring cardiovascular health: mechanistic insights from experimental studies. Clin Sci (Lond) , 123, 53-72.

[32] Dabelea, D, & Pettitt, D. J. (2001). Intrauterine diabetic environment confers risks for type 2 diabetes mellitus and obesity in the offspring, in addition to genetic susceptibility. J Pediatr Endocrinol Metab , 14, 1085-1091.

[33] Dabelea, D, Hanson, R. L, Lindsay, R. S, Pettitt, D. J, Imperatore, G, et al. (2000). Intrauterine exposure to diabetes conveys risks for type 2 diabetes and obesity: a study of discordant sibships. Diabetes , 49, 2208-2211.

[34] Cox, N. J. (1994). Maternal component in NIDDM transmission. How large an effect? Diabetes , 43, 166-168.

[35] Yessoufou, A, & Moutairou, K. (2011). Maternal diabetes in pregnancy: early and long-term outcomes on the offspring and the concept of "metabolic memory". Exp Diabetes Res 2011: 218598.

[36] Clausen, T. D, Mathiesen, E. R, Hansen, T, Pedersen, O, Jensen, D. M, et al. (2009). Overweight and the metabolic syndrome in adult offspring of women with diet-treated gestational diabetes mellitus or type 1 diabetes. J Clin Endocrinol Metab , 94, 2464-2470.

[37] Moore, T. R. (2010). Fetal exposure to gestational diabetes contributes to subsequent adult metabolic syndrome. Am J Obstet Gynecol , 202, 643-649.

[38] Krishnaveni, G. V, Veena, S. R, Hill, J. C, Kehoe, S, Karat, S. C, et al. (2010). Intrauterine exposure to maternal diabetes is associated with higher adiposity and insulin resistance and clustering of cardiovascular risk markers in Indian children. Diabetes Care , 33, 402-404.

[39] Clausen, T. D, Mathiesen, E. R, Hansen, T, Pedersen, O, Jensen, D. M, et al. (2008). High prevalence of type 2 diabetes and pre-diabetes in adult offspring of women

with gestational diabetes mellitus or type 1 diabetes: the role of intrauterine hyperglycemia. Diabetes Care , 31, 340-346.

[40] Silverman, B. L, Metzger, B. E, Cho, N. H, & Loeb, C. A. (1995). Impaired glucose tolerance in adolescent offspring of diabetic mothers. Relationship to fetal hyperinsulinism. Diabetes Care , 18, 611-617.

[41] Plagemann, A, Harder, T, Kohlhoff, R, Rohde, W, & Dorner, G. (1997). Glucose tolerance and insulin secretion in children of mothers with pregestational IDDM or gestational diabetes. Diabetologia , 40, 1094-1100.

[42] Meigs, J. B, Cupples, L. A, & Wilson, P. W. (2000). Parental transmission of type 2 diabetes: the Framingham Offspring Study. Diabetes , 49, 2201-2207.

[43] Boney, C. M, Verma, A, Tucker, R, & Vohr, B. R. (2005). Metabolic syndrome in childhood: association with birth weight, maternal obesity, and gestational diabetes mellitus. Pediatrics 115: e, 290-296.

[44] Wright, C. S, Rifas-shiman, S. L, Rich-edwards, J. W, Taveras, E. M, Gillman, M. W, et al. (2009). Intrauterine exposure to gestational diabetes, child adiposity, and blood pressure. Am J Hypertens , 22, 215-220.

[45] Wu, C. S, Nohr, E. A, Bech, B. H, Vestergaard, M, & Olsen, J. (2012). Long-term health outcomes in children born to mothers with diabetes: a population-based cohort study. PloS One 7: e36727.

[46] Freinkel, N. (1980). Banting Lecture 1980. Of pregnancy and progeny. Diabetes , 29, 1023-1035.

[47] Skilton, M. R. (2008). Intrauterine risk factors for precocious atherosclerosis. Pediatrics , 121, 570-574.

[48] Pinter, E, Haigh, J, Nagy, A, & Madri, J. A. (2001). Hyperglycemia-induced vasculopathy in the murine conceptus is mediated via reductions of VEGF-A expression and VEGF receptor activation. Am J Pathol , 158, 1199-1206.

[49] Torres-farfan, C, Richter, H. G, Germain, A. M, Valenzuela, G. J, Campino, C, et al. (2004). Maternal melatonin selectively inhibits cortisol production in the primate fetal adrenal gland. J Physiol , 554, 841-856.

[50] Fisher, D. (2002). Endocrinology of Fetal Development. Willaims Textbook of Endocrinology. 10th ed: Saunders Editorial. , 811-841.

[51] Benirschke, K, Kaufmann, P, & Baergen, R. N. (2006). Placental types. Pathology of Human Placenta: Springer Editorial. , 30-41.

[52] Talbert, D, & Sebire, N. J. (2004). The dynamic placenta: I. Hypothetical model of a placental mechanism matching local fetal blood flow to local intervillus oxygen delivery. Med Hypotheses , 62, 511-519.

[53] Wang, Y, & Zhao, S. (2010). Vascular biology of the placenta. Morgan & Claypool Life Sciences Editorial.

[54] Cole, L. A. (2009). New discoveries on the biology and detection of human chorionic gonadotropin. Reprod Biol Endocrinol 7: 8.

[55] Armulik, A, Abramsson, A, & Betsholtz, C. (2005). Endothelial/pericyte interactions. Circ Res , 97, 512-523.

[56] Maier, C. L, & Pober, J. S. (2011). Human placental pericytes poorly stimulate and actively regulate allogeneic CD4 T cell responses. Arterioscler Thromb Vasc Biol , 31, 183-189.

[57] Kucuk, M, & Doymaz, F. (2009). Placental weight and placental weight-to-birth weight ratio are increased in diet- and exercise-treated gestational diabetes mellitus subjects but not in subjects with one abnormal value on 100-g oral glucose tolerance test. J Diabetes Complications , 23, 25-31.

[58] Daskalakis, G, Marinopoulos, S, Krielesi, V, Papapanagiotou, A, Papantoniou, N, et al. (2008). Placental pathology in women with gestational diabetes. Acta Obstet Gynecol Scand , 87, 403-407.

[59] Taricco, E, Radaelli, T, & Rossi, G. Nobile de Santis MS, Bulfamante GP, et al. ((2009). Effects of gestational diabetes on fetal oxygen and glucose levels in vivo. BJOG , 116, 1729-1735.

[60] Verma Ranjana MS, Kaul Jagat Mohini (2011). Ultrastructural Changes in the Placental Membrane in Pregnancies Associated with Diabetes. Int J Morphol , 29, 1398-1407.

[61] Dubova, E. A, Pavlov, K. A, Esayan, R. M, Degtyareva, E. I, Shestakova, M. V, et al. (2012). Vascular endothelial growth factor and its receptors in the placenta of women with type 1 diabetes mellitus. Bull Exp Biol Med , 152, 367-370.

[62] Gauster, M, Berghold, V. M, Moser, G, Orendi, K, Siwetz, M, et al. (2011). Fibulin-5 expression in the human placenta. Histochem Cell Biol , 135, 203-213.

[63] Dubova, E. A, Pavlov, K. A, Yesayan, R. M, Nagovitsyna, M. N, Tkacheva, O. N, et al. (2011). Morphometric characteristics of placental villi in pregnant women with diabetes. Bull Exp Biol Med , 151, 650-654.

[64] Jansson, T, Ekstrand, Y, Wennergren, M, & Powell, T. L. (2001). Placental glucose transport in gestational diabetes mellitus. Am J Obstet Gynecol , 184, 111-116.

[65] Osmond, D. T, Nolan, C. J, King, R. G, Brennecke, S. P, & Gude, N. M. (2000). Effects of gestational diabetes on human placental glucose uptake, transfer, and utilisation. Diabetologia , 43, 576-582.

[66] Sciullo, E, Cardellini, G, Baroni, M. G, Torresi, P, Buongiorno, A, et al. (1997). Glucose transporter (Glut1, Glut3) mRNA in human placenta of diabetic and non-diabetic pregnancies. Early Pregnancy , 3, 172-182.

[67] Viau, M, Lafond, J, & Vaillancourt, C. (2009). Expression of placental serotonin transporter and 5-HT 2A receptor in normal and gestational diabetes mellitus pregnancies. Reprod Biomed Online , 19, 207-215.

[68] Jansson, T, Ekstrand, Y, Bjorn, C, Wennergren, M, & Powell, T. L. (2002). Alterations in the activity of placental amino acid transporters in pregnancies complicated by diabetes. Diabetes , 51, 2214-2219.

[69] Schonfelder, G, John, M, Hopp, H, Fuhr, N, Van Der Giet, M, et al. (1996). Expression of inducible nitric oxide synthase in placenta of women with gestational diabetes. FASEB J , 10, 777-784.

[70] Myatt, L. (2010). Review: Reactive oxygen and nitrogen species and functional adaptation of the placenta. Placenta 31 Suppl: S, 66-69.

[71] Madazli, R, Tuten, A, Calay, Z, Uzun, H, Uludag, S, et al. (2008). The incidence of placental abnormalities, maternal and cord plasma malondialdehyde and vascular endothelial growth factor levels in women with gestational diabetes mellitus and nondiabetic controls. Gynecol Obstet Invest , 65, 227-232.

[72] Calderon, I. M, Damasceno, D. C, Amorin, R. L, Costa, R. A, Brasil, M. A, et al. (2007). Morphometric study of placental villi and vessels in women with mild hyperglycemia or gestational or overt diabetes. Diabetes Res Clin Pract , 78, 65-71.

[73] Pietro, L, Daher, S, Rudge, M. V, Calderon, I. M, Damasceno, D. C, et al. (2010). Vascular endothelial growth factor (VEGF) and VEGF-receptor expression in placenta of hyperglycemic pregnant women. Placenta , 31, 770-780.

[74] Leach, L, Babawale, M. O, Anderson, M, & Lammiman, M. (2002). Vasculogenesis, angiogenesis and the molecular organisation of endothelial junctions in the early human placenta. J Vasc Res , 39, 246-259.

[75] Leach, L, Gray, C, Staton, S, Babawale, M. O, Gruchy, A, et al. (2004). Vascular endothelial cadherin and beta-catenin in human fetoplacental vessels of pregnancies complicated by Type 1 diabetes: associations with angiogenesis and perturbed barrier function. Diabetologia , 47, 695-709.

[76] Diab, A. E, Behery, M. M, Ebrahiem, M. A, & Shehata, A. E. (2008). Angiogenic factors for the prediction of pre-eclampsia in women with abnormal midtrimester uterine artery Doppler velocimetry. Int J Gynaecol Obstet , 102, 146-151.

[77] Nicolaides, K. H, Bilardo, C. M, Soothill, P. W, & Campbell, S. (1988). Absence of end diastolic frequencies in umbilical artery: a sign of fetal hypoxia and acidosis. BMJ , 297, 1026-1027.

[78] Madazli, R. (2002). Prognostic factors for survival of growth-restricted fetuses with absent end-diastolic velocity in the umbilical artery. J Perinatol , 22, 286-290.

[79] Skulstad, S. M, Ulriksen, M, Rasmussen, S, & Kiserud, T. (2006). Effect of umbilical ring constriction on Wharton's jelly. Ultrasound Obstet Gynecol , 28, 692-698.

[80] Ghezzi, F, & Raio, L. Di Naro E, Franchi M, Balestreri D, et al. ((2001). Nomogram of Wharton's jelly as depicted in the sonographic cross section of the umbilical cord. Ultrasound Obstet Gynecol , 18, 121-125.

[81] To, W. W, & Mok, C. K. (2009). Fetal umbilical arterial and venous Doppler measurements in gestational diabetic and nondiabetic pregnancies near term. J Matern Fetal Neona Med , 22, 1176-1182.

[82] Ebbing, C, Rasmussen, S, & Kiserud, T. (2011). Fetal hemodynamic development in macrosomic growth. Ultrasound Obstet Gynecol , 38, 303-308.

[83] Farias, M. San Martin R, Puebla C, Pearson JD, Casado JF, et al. (2006). Nitric oxide reduces adenosine transporter ENT1 gene (SLC29A1) promoter activity in human fetal endothelium from gestational diabetes. J Cell Physiol , 208, 451-460.

[84] Wadsack, C, Desoye, G, & Hiden, U. (2012). The feto-placental endothelium in pregnancy pathologies. Wien Med Wochenschr , 162, 220-224.

[85] Escudero, C, & Sobrevia, L. (2008). A hypothesis for preeclampsia: adenosine and inducible nitric oxide synthase in human placental microvascular endothelium. Placenta , 29, 469-483.

[86] Leiva, A, Pardo, F, Ramirez, M. A, Farias, M, Casanello, P, et al. (2011). Fetoplacental vascular endothelial dysfunction as an early phenomenon in the programming of human adult diseases in subjects born from gestational diabetes mellitus or obesity in pregnancy. Exp Diabetes Res 2011: 349286.

[87] Sobrevia, L, Abarzua, F, Nien, J. K, Salomon, C, Westermeier, F, et al. (2011). Review: Differential placental macrovascular and microvascular endothelial dysfunction in gestational diabetes. Placenta 32 Suppl 2: S, 159-164.

[88] Goumans, M. J, & Van Zonneveld, A. J. ten Dijke Transforming growth factor beta-induced endothelial-to-mesenchymal transition: a switch to cardiac fibrosis? Trends Cardiovasc Med 18: 293-298., 2008.

[89] Van Meeteren, L. A. ten Dijke Regulation of endothelial cell plasticity by TGF-beta. Cell Tissue Res 347: 177-186., 2012.

[90] Grant, M. B, Davis, M. I, Caballero, S, Feoktistov, I, Biaggioni, I, et al. (2001). Proliferation, migration, and ERK activation in human retinal endothelial cells through A(2B) adenosine receptor stimulation. Invest Ophthalmol Vis Sci , 42, 2068-2073.

[91] Lang, I, Pabst, M. A, Hiden, U, Blaschitz, A, Dohr, G, et al. (2003). Heterogeneity of microvascular endothelial cells isolated from human term placenta and macrovascular umbilical vein endothelial cells. Eur J Cell Biol , 82, 163-173.

[92] Dye, J, Lawrence, L, Linge, C, Leach, L, Firth, J, et al. (2004). Distinct patterns of microvascular endothelial cell morphology are determined by extracellular matrix composition. Endothelium , 11, 151-167.

[93] Lassance, L, Miedl, H, Konya, V, Heinemann, A, Ebner, B, et al. (2012). Differential response of arterial and venous endothelial cells to extracellular matrix is modulated by oxygen. Histochem Cell Biol. , 137, 641-655.

[94] Escudero, C, & Sobrevia, L. (2009). Understanding physiological significance of high extracellular adenosine levels in feto-placental circulation in preeclamptic pregnancies. In: Sobrevia L, Casanello, P, editor. Membrane Transporters and Receptors in Disease. Kerala, India: Research Signpost. , 27-51.

[95] Hampl, V, Bibova, J, Stranak, Z, Wu, X, Michelakis, E. D, et al. (2002). Hypoxic fetoplacental vasoconstriction in humans is mediated by potassium channel inhibition. Am J Physiol Heart Circ Physiol 283: H, 2440-2449.

[96] Gardner, D. S, Powlson, A. S, & Giussani, D. A. (2001). An in vivo nitric oxide clamp to investigate the influence of nitric oxide on continuous umbilical blood flow during acute hypoxaemia in the sheep fetus. J Physiol , 537, 587-596.

[97] Krause, B. J, Prieto, C. P, & Munoz-urrutia, E. San Martin S, Sobrevia L, et al. (2012). Role of arginase-2 and eNOS in the differential vascular reactivity and hypoxia-induced endothelial response in umbilical arteries and veins. Placenta , 33, 360-366.

[98] Herr, F, Baal, N, Reisinger, K, Lorenz, A, Mckinnon, T, et al. (2007). HCG in the regulation of placental angiogenesis. Results of an in vitro study. Placenta 28 Suppl A: S, 85-93.

[99] Hiden, U, Lang, I, Ghaffari-tabrizi, N, Gauster, M, Lang, U, et al. (2009). Insulin action on the human placental endothelium in normal and diabetic pregnancy. Curr Vasc Pharmacol , 7, 460-466.

[100] San Martin R, Sobrevia L (2006). Gestational diabetes and the adenosine/L-arginine/nitric oxide (ALANO) pathway in human umbilical vein endothelium. Placenta , 27, 1-10.

[101] Guzman-gutierrez, E, Westermeier, F, Salomon, C, Gonzalez, M, Pardo, F, et al. (2012). Insulin-Increased L-Arginine Transport Requires A(2A) Adenosine Receptors Activation in Human Umbilical Vein Endothelium. PloS One 7: e41705.

[102] Casanello, P, Escudero, C, & Sobrevia, L. (2007). Equilibrative nucleoside (ENTs) and cationic amino acid (CATs) transporters: implications in foetal endothelial dysfunction in human pregnancy diseases. Curr Vasc Pharmacol , 5, 69-84.

[103] Rossmanith, W. G, Hoffmeister, U, Wolfahrt, S, Kleine, B, Mclean, M, et al. (1999). Expression and functional analysis of endothelial nitric oxide synthase (eNOS) in human placenta. Mol Hum Reprod , 5, 487-494.

[104] Kossenjans, W, Eis, A, Sahay, R, Brockman, D, & Myatt, L. (2000). Role of peroxynitrite in altered fetal-placental vascular reactivity in diabetes or preeclampsia. Am J Physiol Heart Circ Physiol 278: H, 1311-1319.

[105] Horvath, E. M, Magenheim, R, Kugler, E, Vacz, G, Szigethy, A, et al. (2009). Nitrative stress and poly(ADP-ribose) polymerase activation in healthy and gestational diabetic pregnancies. Diabetologia , 52, 1935-1943.

[106] Salomon, C, Westermeier, F, Puebla, C, Arroyo, P, Guzman-gutierrez, E, et al. (2012). Gestational diabetes reduces adenosine transport in human placental microvascular endothelium, an effect reversed by insulin. PloS One 7: e40578.

[107] Gauster, M, Desoye, G, Totsch, M, & Hiden, U. (2012). The placenta and gestational diabetes mellitus. Curr Diab Rep , 12, 16-23.

[108] Myatt, L, & Cui, X. (2004). Oxidative stress in the placenta. Histochem Cell Biol , 122, 369-382.

[109] Dennery, P. A. (2010). Oxidative stress in development: nature or nurture? Free Radic Biol Med , 49, 1147-1151.

[110] Raijmakers, M. T, Burton, G. J, Jauniaux, E, Seed, P. T, Peters, W. H, et al. (2006). Placental NAD(P)H oxidase mediated superoxide generation in early pregnancy. Placenta , 27, 158-163.

[111] Biri, A, Onan, A, Devrim, E, Babacan, F, Kavutcu, M, et al. (2006). Oxidant status in maternal and cord plasma and placental tissue in gestational diabetes. Placenta , 27, 327-332.

[112] Lappas, M, Hiden, U, Desoye, G, & Froehlich, J. Hauguel-de Mouzon S, et al. (2011). The role of oxidative stress in the pathophysiology of gestational diabetes mellitus. Antioxid Redox Signal , 15, 3061-3100.

[113] Villalobos, R C. P, Cabrera, L, Palma, C, Rojas, S, Gallardo, V, & González, M. (2012). High D-glucose increases the NADPH oxidase 2 and 4 mRNA levels and synthesis of reactive oxygen species involving the activity of PKC and 38MAPK in HUVEC.. Proc Physiol Soc 27: [Abstract].

[114] Quagliaro, L, Piconi, L, Assaloni, R, Martinelli, L, Motz, E, et al. (2003). Intermittent high glucose enhances apoptosis related to oxidative stress in human umbilical vein endothelial cells: the role of protein kinase C and NAD(P)H-oxidase activation. Diabetes , 52, 2795-2804.

[115] Frohlich, J. D, Huppertz, B, Abuja, P. M, Konig, J, & Desoye, G. (2012). Oxygen modulates the response of first-trimester trophoblasts to hyperglycemia. Am J Pathol , 180, 153-164.

[116] Jirkovska, M, Kucera, T, Kalab, J, Jadrnicek, M, Niedobova, V, et al. (2012). The branching pattern of villous capillaries and structural changes of placental terminal villi in type 1 diabetes mellitus. Placenta , 33, 343-351.

[117] Higgins, M, Felle, P, Mooney, E. E, Bannigan, J, & Mcauliffe, F. M. (2011). Stereology of the placenta in type 1 and type 2 diabetes. Placenta , 32, 564-569.

[118] Mayhew, T. M. (2002). Enhanced fetoplacental angiogenesis in pre-gestational diabetes mellitus: the extra growth is exclusively longitudinal and not accompanied by microvascular remodelling. Diabetologia , 45, 1434-1439.

[119] Mayhew, T. M, Sorensen, F. B, Klebe, J. G, & Jackson, M. R. (1994). Growth and maturation of villi in placentae from well-controlled diabetic women. Placenta , 15, 57-65.

[120] Jirkovska, M, Kubinova, L, Janacek, J, Moravcova, M, Krejci, V, et al. (2002). Topological properties and spatial organization of villous capillaries in normal and diabetic placentas. J Vasc Res , 39, 268-278.

[121] Jauniaux, E, & Burton, G. J. (2006). Villous histomorphometry and placental bed biopsy investigation in Type I diabetic pregnancies. Placenta , 27, 468-474.

[122] Kolluru, G. K, Bir, S. C, & Kevil, C. G. (2012). Endothelial dysfunction and diabetes: effects on angiogenesis, vascular remodeling, and wound healing. Int J Vasc Med 2012: 918267.

[123] Penno, G, Pucci, L, Lucchesi, D, Lencioni, C, Iorio, M. C, et al. (2011). Circulating endothelial progenitor cells in women with gestational alterations of glucose tolerance. Diab Vasc Dis Res , 8, 202-210.

[124] Acosta, J. C, Haas, D. M, Saha, C. K, Dimeglio, L. A, Ingram, D. A, et al. (2011). Gestational diabetes mellitus alters maternal and neonatal circulating endothelial progenitor cell subsets. Am J Obstet Gynecol 204: 254 ee215., 258-254.

[125] Ettelaie, C, Su, S, Li, C, & Collier, M. E. (2008). Tissue factor-containing microparticles released from mesangial cells in response to high glucose and AGE induce tube formation in microvascular cells. Microvasc Res , 76, 152-160.

[126] Helske, S, Vuorela, P, Carpen, O, Hornig, C, Weich, H, et al. (2001). Expression of vascular endothelial growth factor receptors 1, 2 and 3 in placentas from normal and complicated pregnancies. Mol Hum Reprod , 7, 205-210.

[127] Janota, J, Pomyje, J, Toth, D, Sosna, O, Zivny, J, et al. (2003). Expression of angiopoietic factors in normal and type-I diabetes human placenta: a pilot study. Eur J Obstet Gynecol Reprod Biol , 111, 153-156.

[128] Hiden, U, Maier, A, Bilban, M, Ghaffari-tabrizi, N, Wadsack, C, et al. (2006). Insulin control of placental gene expression shifts from mother to foetus over the course of pregnancy. Diabetologia , 49, 123-131.

[129] Escudero, C, Puebla, C, Westermeier, F, & Sobrevia, L. (2009). Potential cell signalling mechanisms involved in differential placental angiogenesis in mild and severe preeclampsia. Curr Vasc Pharmacol , 7, 475-485.